introducing research and evidence-based practice for nurses

Jeremy Jolley

PEARSON

Harlow, England • London • New York • ... • Singapore • Hong Kong
Tokyo • Seoul • Taipei • New Delhi • C... • Munich • Paris • Milan

Pearson Education Limited
Edinburgh Gate
Harlow
Essex CM20 2JE
England

and Associated Companies throughout the world

Visit us on the World Wide Web at:
www.pearsoned.co.uk

First published 2010

ISBN: 978-0-273-71916-8

British Library Cataloguing-in-Publication Data
A catalogue record for this book is available from the British Library

Library of Congress Cataloging-in-Publication Data

Jolley, Jeremy,
  Introducing research and evidence-based practice for nurses / Jeremy Jolley.
      p. ; cm.
  Includes bibliographical references and index.
  ISBN 978-0-273-71916-8 (pbk.)
  1. Nursing--Research. 2. Evidence-based nursing. I. Title.
  [DNLM: 1. Nursing Research. 2. Evidence-Based Nursing. WY 20.5 J75i
2010]
  RT81.5.J65 2010
  610.73072--dc22

                            2009032269

10 9 8 7 6 5 4 3 2 1
14 13 12 11 10

Typeset in 10.25/14pt Interstate Light by 30
Printed in Great Britain by Henry Ling Ltd., at the Dorset Press, Dorchester, Dorset.

The publisher's policy is to use paper manufactured from sustainable forests.

To Susan, Alice and Catherine

Contents

Preface

This book has been written for the student who is new to research and evidence-based practice. The book's aim is to help the many nursing students who struggle to understand what research in nursing is all about. Of course, there are already lots of books on nursing research. There are big books, complicated books, books that try but fail to summarise the whole subject of research. There are lots of books, and many are tedious, stuffy and incomprehensible to those new to the subject. This book is different: it deals only with the important aspects of nursing research, what students need to know for research to begin to make real sense. This book isn't stuffy, because stuffy is boring and life is too short for such non-sense. Real research is exciting, it is imagining something new, it is dealing with real-life questions and finding answers, it is making nursing better for real patients and real nurses.

Research can sometimes look complex and perplexing, it can make students feel unintelligent and lost, it can make students feel stupid or make them reject research altogether. This book aims to put that right, to show the reader that research can be understood, that research is at its core really simple and genuinely useful. All students are clever and no one gets this far in their nursing programme without possessing real vigour and enthusiasm for the subject they have chosen to study and to practise. We should all believe in students: nursing will soon be their responsibility and they will need an understanding of research and evidence-based practice to ensure that nursing continues to grow and to develop.

Nursing students often don't get the opportunity to experience research, to work on a real research project. This lack of a practice element to their studies makes it hard for them to understand what research is all about. Nursing students are often asked to evaluate a piece of nursing research, without having any experience of research themselves. This last is akin to asking them to watch a neurosurgeon at work and then to evaluate how well the surgery was performed. Furthermore, nursing is a particularly broad discipline and, as a result of this, it employs almost every kind of research strategy that exists. Nursing uses quantitative and qualitative approaches to research; it uses everything from surveys to experiments to approaches that seek one person's understanding of another at the deepest psychological and emotional level.

The richness and diversity of nursing research leave other disciplines standing, but they also mean that it is much more difficult for nursing students to get to grips with research. How much easier it is for the average medical student, who can be content to know the meaning of a double-blind trial. Let us be perfectly clear: there is a lot to nursing research. It is sad that so very few existing texts try to help the nursing student through this maze. This book is different: it aims to provide just such guidance, to hold the student's hand through the journey of discovery. The book does this, while consistently valuing the subject matter for its central importance to nursing, for the intelligence of each and every student and for the potential each student carries with them to produce real advances in patient care.

Acknowledgements

We would like to thank the reviewers for their comments:

Amy Dopson, University of Surrey
Ted Hewitt, University of York
Dr Khim Horton, University of Surrey
Neil A. Jones, University of Central Lancashire

We are grateful to the following for permission to reproduce copyright material:

Figures 2.1, 2.2, 2.3 © EBSCO Publishing, Inc., 2009. All rights reserved; Figure 5.1 from *Wong's Essentials of Pediatric Nursing*, 7th ed., Mosby: St Louis (Hockenberry, M.J., Wilson, D., and Wilkelstein, M.L. 2005) p. 1259. Used with permission, Copyright, Mosby.

In some instances we have been unable to trace the owners of copyright material, and we would appreciate any information that would enable us to do so.

Chapter 1
Research is simple

Chapter outline

Students often find it difficult to understand the real meaning of the terms 'research' and 'evidence-based practice' . This chapter aims to make it possible for anyone to understand what these terms mean and why they are relevant to nursing and to health care. In short, this chapter will help you make sense of what can sometimes seem a complex area of study. Research can seem to be complex, but this chapter will show you that research is really very simple. Indeed, this chapter will convince you that you already know about research.

What is research?

You are probably reading this because you have been asked to study research or evidence-based practice. Perhaps you have been asked to write your first research proposal. Research can seem complex, but it is actually little more than what you already do and what you already know. Fundamentally, research is simple and this book aims to keep it that way.

Research is relevant to you and it is relevant to nursing. In fact, research and nursing are inseparable. Nursing needs to be questioning, nursing needs to be seeking to find better ways to help people, nursing needs research. Nursing research is similar to the questioning and investigative stance that clinical nurses adopt all of the time. Think about it: when you admit a patient or client to the clinical area, you will want to talk with them, watch them and ask them questions. Your assessment of this patient isn't haphazard or random; it is organised, it is systematic. This systematic approach to the gathering of information is not only similar to research; it is what *defines* research. Research is not just any old haphazard collection of data; research is organised, thought-through and systematised – exactly like your assessment of a new patient. Furthermore, in your practice of nursing you will use skills that are identical to the skills used in research. You will, for example, try to collect data that are rich enough (sufficient enough) for your purpose, and you will use data-collection methods that are purposeful and thought-through – just as in a research project. When you admit a new patient, you use a face-to-face interview; you do not give them a questionnaire or get them involved in a focus group. So it is with research: research uses the most appropriate means of data collection, and that may be and often is exactly the technique you use when admitting a new patient.

Nursing students do sometimes become confused about research. They find that they are unsure about what research is. Now we know why they are confused. Research is what nursing is, and nursing is what research is. No wonder students are confused: they are looking for something new to study when in fact they have been living and breathing it since the first day of their course.

New words

Data (Datum) Values or factual information collected during research. Note that 'data' is plural, so that a researcher might say 'these data are interesting'. The singular form is 'datum'.

You already know about research; it is in every fibre of your enquiring mind and you can use it to contribute to nursing and make things better.

Let us be clear: you are studying research because you have a lively and intelligent mind; in fact, you have already acquired so much knowledge of research that you will not find your present studies difficult. Indeed, you already know most of the important principles of research.

You may be concerned that you are not very good at mathematics; well, that's no problem. Researchers need only to use computer applications that deal with numbers, as a word processor deals with words. Don't worry if you are not good with numbers. Many researchers are not good with numbers either.

There are lots of definitions of research, so let's discard them all and start again. Have a look at the definitions listed in Table 1.1.

Table 1.1 Definitions of research

Scientific method	The scientific method is a sort of philosophical underpinning for everything we call science. It is very similar to the nursing process in that it is systematic and objective. It goes something like this:
	1. The hunch (a gut feeling about a possible enquiry)
	2. Literature review to find out what is already known
	3. Problem identification
	4. The hypothesis
	5. Plan for research
	6. Data collection
	7. Data analysis
	8. Discussion of results/evaluation
Research	Research is any enquiry that is systematic in its approach and that seeks to ensure that the results of the enquiry cannot be criticised on the grounds of poor technique
Evidence-based practice	Evidence-based practice is said to exist where there is a clear attempt to base clinical practice upon known evidence. Research evidence is usually the best form of evidence, but sometimes other forms of evidence are used

Figure 1.1 shows the relationship between three important concepts. In nursing, the purpose of science and of research is to produce practice that is based on evidence; that is, practice that is understood and is known to be effective.

Figure 1.1 Relationship between three important concepts in nursing

New words

Robust A word that means 'solid' or 'unshakable' and that is applied to research studies that are difficult to criticise.

So, what *is* research? Research is nothing more than systematic enquiry. It is an endeavour to discover new information, in a manner that is structured, systematic and objective, while using techniques (methodologies) that are robust. All researchers want to produce research of good quality (research that is robust). If the methodology is questionable, so will be the results. The definition of research given here applies to all research, from that which takes place in laboratories, to that which focuses on human experiences. All research is just a systematic enquiry.

The 'salt bath' and poor methodology

Nurses are good at using sound principles for the collection of data. However, occasionally those sound principles have not been well applied. The history of the salt bath is interesting because it warns us to be on our guard against poor methodologies.

Through most of the twentieth century, salt baths were used to help heal wounds. Patients could often be found relaxing in baths to which had been added a variable amount of table salt (Austin 1988). It had long been argued that salt baths were more or less essential for wound healing to take place.

Now, let us prove that salt baths do work. Let's do an experiment. The next time you cut your finger, put it into a cup of water with salt in it (it doesn't matter how much salt). Do this three times a day (because 'three times a day' sounds very therapeutic). Your finger will get better. So, salt baths work; we have proved it.

Of course, you will have seen that our methodology is less than robust. The chances are that your finger would have got better without the salt-water treatment. Wounds have a tendency to get better all on their own. The problem here is that we did not set up a control. If we had tested, say, 50 cut fingers given no treatment and 50 cut fingers given a saline bath, then we would find that being dipped in saline three times a day made no difference whatsoever to the healing rate or the incidence of successful healing.

However, before we criticise nurses in the past for their lack of research (see Walsh and Ford 1989), we should bear in mind that nursing is a big discipline containing a great deal of expertise. We are all human and it is difficult to question practices that are long-established and widely accepted. When you next go to work, take a look at what you find yourself doing and ask 'What exactly is the evidence that this works?'

Research – a two-headed beast

It will probably not surprise you that there is more than one form of research. You are probably aware that a survey, for example, is not the same thing as an experiment. Research does come in several different forms. For the moment, however, it would be useful to introduce the two main research variants. Arguably, every research study will fit into one or other of these two variants:

- *Quantitative research*: this deals in quantities of things. The data from quantitative studies exist usually in the form of numbers, which can then be quantified (added up) and subjected to statistical analysis.

- *Qualitative research*: this deals in the quality of things. However, this definition is not very helpful. In practice, this category of research deals in data that exist as words and concepts rather than as numbers.

Example from the literature and research

Meyers *et al.* (2004) used a quantitative approach to study the experience of family members being present during invasive procedures and resuscitation. It was found that family members were positive about their experience and considered being present as their right. There was found to be no evidence of psychological trauma to family members who stayed with their loved one during resuscitation. The study found that nurses and senior doctors tended to be in favour of family members being present with the patient, but junior doctors tend to be less happy. Perhaps nurses and senior doctors are more confident about the care they provide during invasive procedures and resuscitation than are junior doctors and are thus more willing to be watched at a time when nursing and medical skills are critical to the patient's survival.

Example from the literature and research

Wigert *et al.* (2006) conducted a qualitative study into mothers' experience of their newborn child being in intensive care. Using interviews with mothers, it was found that the mother often felt excluded from the social environment of the unit and that this then had a negative effect on her maternal feelings toward her own baby. The implications of this study are that staff should make mothers feel welcome and should help mothers to feel valued and useful. This will not only make mothers feel better about themselves but will also enable them to develop a normal and warm relationship with their child.

These two categories almost represent fields of research, with researchers often spending their whole career in one field or the other. Nursing is a little unusual in making use of both forms and even mixing the two approaches together within the same study (Canning *et al.* 2007). This mixing of these two approaches is an example of nursing leading research and of it being prepared to 'think outside the box'.

You already know about research

Research is essentially a simple activity. However, research often looks complex and research studies can be quite large. Research is simple but it possesses its own language, which can take time to learn. Research uses a range of techniques to ensure that the resulting data are what they are meant to be and not biased or unreliable. These techniques can look complex at first, but they are not complex. Then there are those numbers: statistical analyses can look very complex. However, appearances are deceptive and the most advanced and apparently complex statistic will always be simple and intuitive at its core. Furthermore, it is the principles of research that you should learn now. For example, by the end of this book, you will understand the rationale for using inferential statistics, but you will not need to learn how to calculate every single statistical procedure. With these principles in your pocket, you will know all you need to know about research and, indeed, you will be ready to use research in your own area of clinical practice.

Research is systematic enquiry and is something with which you are already very familiar. Say that you are looking for material for an essay on the management of post-surgery pain. You go to the library and you go to the section on pain management and then perhaps to the section on surgery. You might do an electronic literature search using the keywords 'surgery' and 'pain'. Finally, you might go and have a word with one of the faculty staff members who has done some work in this area. That's good. You have undertaken a search, but not just any old search: your search has been goal-orientated and systematic. You didn't look in the history of art section of the library; nor did you ask that student who keeps failing her essay for help. You thought about it, not wanting to waste your time. You wanted to be focused, to be clear about what you were looking for. There is no material difference between this and research.

Perhaps you think that research is more complex because it often includes experiments, difficult language and lots of numbers. Not at all; in fact, you used a library - and lots of people can't do that. You used an electronic search engine - most people can't do that. Importantly, you used a goal-orientated and systematic approach - hardly anyone can do that (just watch MPs in the House of Commons trying to decide something). The fact is, you are brilliant, a real achiever, a star. Seriously, you are a very clever person. In fact, you already do research and what there is left to learn will come easily and intuitively.

What has research to do with nursing?

Student nurses at the beginning of their programme of study are often surprised to discover that they are expected to learn about research. When asked why they wish to be nurses, many interviewees will say that they want to make a difference to peoples' lives by doing something to help in times of illness or distress. Interviewees will often indicate that they are practical people with a gift for getting on with others and that they want to do a socially useful job. It would be unusual in the extreme to come across a candidate who wanted to enter nursing because of a desire to research or to spend their time in academia.

The fact that newcomers to the profession are sometimes surprised to learn even that there is such a thing as nursing research probably has something to do with the image of research and the image of nursing. When you have a moment, use your computer to search for images of research. You will find pictures of men and women in white coats peering into microscopes, rows of test tubes in laboratories, and complex flow diagrams covered with tiny writing. Now look for images of nurses. You will find pictures of uniformed men and women dealing with sick people in hospital. These images will be of nurses doing clinical things such as taking blood-pressure readings and helping people to walk (while invariably smiling). The words 'nursing' and 'research' seem to have little in common. Of course, it just takes a moment's reflection to realise that these are very simplistic depictions of both research and nursing, but in a way that's precisely the point: there is more to both nursing and research than there might first appear to be. Research, for example, does not always use expensive equipment in hi-tech laboratories. Sometimes, researchers will collect information using a method based on something we can all do: speaking to another person and listening carefully to what they say in response. Equally, the variety and complexity of nursing are not easily or accurately represented by the familiar stereotypes of paper caps, crisp uniforms and hospital beds.

Practical nursing and research – the same motivation

Why do you turn up for work in the morning? Initially, nursing students are often motivated by a desire to help and support other people in practical ways (Rognstad and Aasland 2007); this is probably true of you. We need to look no further than this to find a major source of motivation for quite a lot of nursing research. Most of the nursing research that you will read about in journals and textbooks will have been undertaken by nurses. Some of these nurses will have done the research while working in a clinical role, while some research will have been carried out by nurses working as teachers and researchers in university departments of nursing; but nearly all of it will have been done by people with a nursing qualification. People don't stop being nurses when they become researchers: the motivation that led them to the nursing profession is the same motivation that leads them to undertake and publish research projects. You can see this by turning to a journal and looking at the titles of the articles that are published there to get a sense of what they are about. The subjects that are being investigated will often relate to everyday nursing problems and concerns.

Why knowledge can't simply be passed on from one person to another

Nurses, in their everyday work, try to help people to solve problems related to their health. Sometimes problems are entirely unique to one particular individual, while at other times they fall into patterns. For example, it's very common for patients to experience pain in various circumstances, and nurses will want to relieve this if they can; and although each person's pain is unique in the sense that they are the only person who can feel it, experienced nurses learn that peoples' stories of pain tend to have common features, not least of which is that pain is generally considered to be unpleasant. As nurses build up a bank of experience, they may try a number of different ways of addressing these problems, some of which seem to work at least some of the time, while others are rather less useful. On occasion they may resort to traditional approaches that they have learned from other nurses, and again they may have variable rates of success as they use these methods. One of the problems of working on your own or in a small team is that you can build up what we might call 'customary' ways of working. Certain habits of practice develop. The problem is that it can be very difficult for an individual nurse, or a small group of nurses working together on a ward, to get an objective sense of the effectiveness of what they are doing.

Here is an account by a lecturer in nursing, looking back at his early experience as a student nurse:

> One of my first experiences as a student nurse was to be shown a traditional way of caring for a patient with a pressure sore. The patient was a man with advanced multiple sclerosis, and he had a sore the size of a 10p coin on his bottom. The ward sister showed me how to roll the patient on to his side, and then used a brush to apply beaten egg white to the sore. Next, she used a plastic tube to blow oxygen on to the egg white to dry it.

> I was a bit surprised at this treatment and asked the sister what benefit it was. She explained that pressure sores occurred when tissue was poorly nourished and badly oxygenated. Thus, there was clearly a logic to what she was doing, though looking back I suspect that the simple act of turning the patient on to his side for a while was of more use than the egg white and oxygen.

In recent years, nurse researchers have investigated many traditional treatments of this kind and found that they simply don't work (Helberg *et al.* 2006). Research is a way of testing our practice and finding out which approaches are most effective. This is sometimes known as clinical effectiveness.

There is a lot of nursing knowledge out there and nurses know how to do a lot of things. A nurse, can, for example, pick up a copy of the current European Resuscitation Council guidelines (Baskett and Zideman 2005), read them and know what to do when someone needs to be resuscitated. In the same way, there exists a plethora of textbooks that the enquiring nurse can use to guide practice. So, why is there a need for research? Why not wait until all the research becomes incorporated into the textbooks and then just read the textbooks?

If you wait for this to happen, you are not participating in your profession. It's like waiting for someone to cook your dinner and then waiting for someone else to do the washing up. You are just sitting on the couch getting fat. Nursing is *your* discipline: it isn't run for you, you are running it. There isn't anyone to do the washing up: you have to do it. If you want to eat, you have to cook your own dinner. Nursing belongs to you. As a nurse, you have a responsibility to make things better, to take things forward, to improve the service that nurses offer patients. What we know now is not good enough; it can never be good enough because it can be even better. Your job is to make it better, and research is the key way to make that happen. It is in this way that nursing is a profession. If it were just a job, you could indeed wait for someone to tell you what to do. Nursing isn't just a job: nurses have a responsibility not only to their patients and not only to their shift and to their hospital or team but also to their profession. It is not good enough that you provide expert care only to your patient; you must also provide expert care, research and leadership to the whole profession.

Patients and others who depend on nurses should be certain that 'their' nurse is doing more than obeying orders or following the guidelines found in text-books. From the most junior student to the nurse consultant, nurses need to be aware of research and aware of the gaps in research where we are still igno-rant of how best to help patients. However, even this is not enough: every nurse should be capable of addressing the gaps in our knowledge and of seek-ing out ways to increase our understanding, so that nurses everywhere are better able to provide the best care that is possible.

Nursing is a practice discipline

New words

Theory A mature set of interrelated ideas supported by at least some evidence. In time, even well-developed theory may be shown to be wrong.

Inductive research Research raised from questions about practice rather than from theory. Inductive research can be used to generate new theory, but it usually exists to answer gaps in our knowledge.

Deductive research Research that is derived from theory. This is unusual in nursing but more common in psychology, where, for example, one might speak of 'psychoanalytical research' (research that stems from psychoanalytical theory).

Nursing is a practice discipline; nursing has no purpose beyond its practice. For this reason, nursing research is almost wholly inductive; that is, it seeks to answer questions about practice. Nursing does not have a well-defined concept-base; there are no real theories of nursing as there are theoretical perspectives in psychology, such as Freudian theory and behaviourism. Nursing research does not, on the whole, seek to produce either theory or pure knowledge as do disci-plines such as psychology and sociology. Nursing is a practice discipline and as such does not seek to produce either knowledge or theory for its own sake; rather, it seeks to push back the frontiers of nursing practice.

There is a study element to research. However, there is a study element to the life of every professional person. Learning is a life-long process in any profes-sion. The student who thinks that three years of study will set them up for a lifetime of practice is misguided.

So, yes, there is a study element to research. One has to learn how to find research and then how to read it, interpret it, practise it and implement research into practice. Get used to the idea, for it is common to professional life. For a full professional life, there must be study and practice. Research in nursing is almost always directed at questions of practice and is purposed to improve the work of all nurses for the benefit of the patient.

Where is research?

Nursing research can sometimes seem invisible, but it is present and is eminently practical in nature. When you first started nursing, you probably found it all a little confusing. You had to find the ward then the ward office. Later on, you struggled to find the nasogastric tubes and the dermatology department. For a while, it was confusing. Eventually, however, you worked out where everything was and you began to feel at home in your clinical environment. Perhaps you have come to feel a sense of mastery over it all and you can now be found telling more junior students what to do and where to go to find things. However, research may be something that you have never really managed to make much sense of. After all, where is it? Where is the research department? Ages ago, you worked out what dermatology is, but what is research? Surely any self-respecting thing ought at least to be visible? So it is that you may have relegated research to the weird and ephemeral, like nursing theory and philosophy. After all, if research was real, you would see the staff practising it and talking about it; it would have become part of what you do.

The truth is that, for many practitioners, research is something other people do; for many practitioners, research is indeed weird and ephemeral. You will have asked yourself how this could be. More importantly, you will have asked why you are being asked to study research when there are lots of other, more practical things that you could be learning. The fact is that nursing is a developing discipline. What you see around you is not what nursing was 30 years ago and it is not what nursing will be in 30 years' time. Nursing is in the process of developing into a fully fledged profession. It has come a long way but there is still a distance to be travelled. Nursing is developing into a research-orientated profession but it is not there yet. So it is that your programme of study is preparing you not for the past, and not even for today, but for your practice tomorrow.

Nursing cannot afford to stand still. It must always be searching for better ways of caring for people and it should never be satisfied with the ways things are now. So, your course should not fit exactly with what you see nurses doing in practice. You are the future of nursing and you are learning to practise in the future. When you first started nursing, you probably wanted to be just like the other nurses, you wanted to be an accepted member of the team, to know the routine and to look and feel like a nurse. That is as it should be, but sooner or later you will have to learn how to be yourself, to be your own sort of nurse and to imprint yourself on the future of nursing. You have seen the staff and tried to be like them. However, the time will come when you will have to create the future of nursing from your unique skills and your enthusiasm to make things better. Research is about moving things forward, rather than learning what other people already know.

Let us leave nursing for a moment and look at the disciplines of psychology and medicine; let's see if we can find research there. Psychology is split broadly into two career pathways, clinical psychology and academic psychology. Most psychology research is conducted by academic psychologists working in universities. So psychology students have no difficulty working out where to find research: as they go though their programme of study, research will be all around them.

So where is research in medicine? You know that there is research in medicine. You will have heard about the struggle to cure diseases for which treatment is still largely ineffective. You will have heard of research that led to the development of vaccines for such diseases as smallpox and poliomyelitis, which once wrought death and grief on a massive scale. If you work in a large teaching hospital you will even find that there are medical research departments. Your hospital might have a cardiac research department, for example. However, smaller hospitals often lack these research departments, so why is this? Most medical research takes place in universities. The larger teaching hospitals are staffed by the very same medical people who work in the universities and so you see research taking place there. However, in the non-teaching hospitals, the medical staff do not tend to have academic posts and so less research is carried out. The medical staff in smaller hospitals are a bit like the nurses you have worked with: for them, research is largely something other people do. However, all doctors and all nurses take seriously their responsibility to ensure their practice is grounded in current research.

So neither medicine nor nursing is perfect, but remember that you are learning to work in the future, not the present. The influence of research is growing very quickly. Even today, there are many practitioners for whom research is a central part of their working lives. Research is all around them and they live and breathe research every day. Suggest to any of these people that research is dry, academic and hard to define and they will look at you as if you have come from another planet. If they should have sufficient patience with you, they will pause and explain that research is anything but dry and academic. They will tell you that research is eminently practical, it is logically construed and orientated to finding answers to the everyday problems of clinical practice. Ask them to show you a researcher and you will be shown someone with their sleeves rolled up, doing work that could not be regarded as anything other than practical and pragmatic. If you thought that research was dry and academic, or ill-defined and nebulous, you were wrong.

So research is a very practical craft. It is, in fact, at the practical end of practice; it is more practical than is most of nursing. So you asked the professor of nursing to show you a researcher and you were shown a real person doing seriously practical work. You asked the researcher what was involved in the work and what was the goal of it and you received a brief and plain reply. The work of the researcher is practical and clearly understood.

The role of research in practical nursing

Let's think of an imaginary example of the role research plays in everyday nursing:

> *Joe is a lively nine-year-old who loves to play football in his school team. One day he jumps to head a ball but accidentally collides with the goal post and cuts his head. The cut is about 2 cm long and there is blood all over the place. Joe's parents take him to the accident and emergency department of the local hospital. A nurse makes an initial assessment. The nurse asks Joe how he cut his head and asks his parents whether he lost consciousness. She then uses glue to stick the edges of the wound together before sending Joe and his parents home.*

This is a brief description of a simple event. Things like this happen every day and will be very familiar to any nurse with accident and emergency experience. However, you may be surprised to learn just how much of the interaction is shaped by the findings of research.

Children can have a serious and life-threatening head injury without having a fractured skull and with very little bruising. However, nurses know how to determine whether a child is likely to have a minor or a serious head injury: they consider prognostic indicators such as those identified by Kieslich *et al.* (2001). If nurses based their practice on experience alone, then it would take them hundreds of years to learn what prognostic indicators could be used effectively.

Dealing with Joe's wound may be both frightening and painful. The nurse may decide to use distraction to help Joe deal effectively with the investigation and treatment of his wound. However, the nurse will want to use a form of distraction that is known to be reliable and so he or she chooses to base this practice on research such as that by Windich-Biermeier *et al.* (2007). This study demonstrates that when performed properly, distraction can be a valuable tool in helping children cope with fearful and painful procedures.

The glue that the nurse uses to close Joe's wound will have been chosen for its effectiveness. All glues sting a little, but research has demonstrated which glues are maximally effective while causing the least discomfort to children (Charters 2000).

As you watch this nurse in action, you might be forgiven for thinking that he or she is simply doing what is common sense or perhaps what he or she has been trained to do. You look at the nurse, quietly and competently helping Joe; you do not see the research. However, in this simple scenario, research is everywhere. The nurse's actions are guided at almost every step by research.

This little example has begun to illustrate some of the reasons for nurses' involvement in research and to show why nurses are expected to learn about research and to apply the findings in their practice when they become qualified practitioners. We have already made the point that people are often surprised by the extent and importance of nursing research because they imagine, quite wrongly, that practice and research are two entirely different things.

Who does research today?

Just as research itself can be hidden from the world of nursing practice, so too can be the people who carry out research. Most nursing research is probably undertaken by nurses who work in universities. However, we have noted that nursing research has a practice focus and the studies that take place tend to involve practice areas, patients, clients and nursing staff.

Research tends to be expensive: people's time costs money and research projects can take a long time to complete. The agencies providing research funding need to make sure that their funds are used wisely – so funding tends to go to research teams that have a known history of producing good research. These research teams are likely to reside in one or more universities. However, those who fund research will usually want to see evidence of collaboration with the practice setting and, because of this, there are opportunities for practice staff to become involved in research – so most good research is managed by university staff in close collaboration with clinical staff. There are important exceptions to this, but it is still the case that the universities do and will continue to play a central role in the conduct of research studies.

As a nursing student, you stand with one foot in the university and one foot in practice. You will probably see your future in practice and you look forward to the day when you will have both of your feet in the practice setting. It may be wise, however, to consider maintaining your links with your university. Nursing research is as much a part of nursing as medical research is part of medicine. This is a difficult but important idea to accept, especially for the student who may see their passage through the university as transient and self-limiting. In fact, nursing is a life-long-learning profession, and a nurse's relationship with the university should not end when they graduate. You will never stop having ideas about how nursing could be improved, and it is sometimes good to share those ideas with university staff so that nursing can be developed to improve the care provided to patients and clients. This is rightly a bilateral relationship. Nurses in practice know where they are frustrated by an inability to provide the patient or client with what is needed. University staff have the research expertise to develop a study that could move our knowledge forward. This collaboration of equal partners is an effective model for the building of research projects for the improvement of nursing care.

The message is clear: when you leave university, don't leave. If you have left university, go back. This does not mean that you should go back to undertake another course of study but that you should go back to maintain effective liaisons with academic staff. In this way, ideas are shared, projects are started, and the boundaries of nursing and of science are pushed back – by nurses, by people like you.

Try this: Go to the Dean of your faculty or search out one of the professors – go on, corner them! Ask them for a list of ongoing research taking place within the faculty. List those research projects in the space provided on p. 17. You may be surprised just how much research activity is going on all around you.

(1) _____ (10) _____

(2) _____ (11) _____

(3) _____ (12) _____

(4) _____ (13) _____

(5) _____ (14) _____

(6) _____ (15) _____

(7) _____ (16) _____

(8) _____ (17) _____

(9) _____ (18) _____

So, now you know what the staff are doing when they are not teaching you, having lunch, having coffee, going for an ice cream, going home early, coming to work late, phoning their partner, having a drink in the bar, reading the newspaper in the library, snoozing in the office, surfing the Web for a new car, collecting their post, collecting their post again, chatting to the receptionist, reading another paper in the library ...

Now do one last thing: choose one of the studies taking place in your faculty, from the list you made above – select something that looks interesting. Go and see the person in charge of this project (he or she may be in the library reading a newspaper) and get them to tell you about their project. Now don't take 'no' for an answer – insist on a meeting with them (they have read that newspaper twice anyway). Get the following details about their study:

- The title

- The duration of the project

- What the study aims to achieve

- How the study relates to the practice of nursing.

So, we have noted that most research is undertaken within universities but in close collaboration with clinical staff. It is unfortunate that a lot of research is invisible to the casual observer, even to students. However, if you just ask, you will find that research is already everywhere.

Research: what's in it for me?

There are two main reasons why people become involved in research:

- To push forward the frontiers of science

- To push forward the frontiers of their career.

These two goals do not have to be in conflict. However, the acceptance of research in nursing is sometimes limited by the belief that researchers are simply furthering their own career. Think about it, though: how many wealthy researchers do you know? No one ever made a fortune out of nursing research. Furthermore, it is no bad thing to want to progress one's career. Take a look at the nurses you meet in your clinical area; some of them will be happy to do what they are doing now until they retire. That's good because good nursing needs good experience. However, look around you again; in fact, go and search out those nurses who have progressed their career and talk to them about it. Go and talk with your nurse manager and with a nurse practitioner or nurse consultant. Here are some questions you can ask them:

- Why did you want to be anything other than a ward nurse?

....

- At what point did you realise that you wanted to progress your career?

....

- How can you contribute more now that you are in your present role?

....

Being involved in research is one way in which nurses can contribute more. A ward or community nurse does a great job; it is the job to which you probably and rightly aspire. However, nurses are not static creatures but find that they are able to deliver more as they gain experience, skills and knowledge. When you qualify and begin to work as a ward or community nurse, you will be doing a fantastic job. That job will be uniquely practical and intellectual, and it will be rewarding on many different levels. However, it won't be easy: you have chosen one of the most difficult programmes of study ever offered by universities, and you are looking forward to doing a job that will tax every fibre of your body, mind and soul. It is precisely this sense of endeavour, this willingness to do more than what is easy and comfortable, that will drive you on to do more and more with your career. Importantly, you will come to a point in your career when you can deliver expert patient care. It is at that point that you will want to begin to influence not only what you can do but what all nurses can do. At this point, you will want to make a difference not only to one or two patients but to many patients.

As a ward or community nurse, you will find yourself addressing this question: How can I ensure that this patient's pain is controlled more capably? Sooner or later, you will find yourself asking: How can nurses better manage patients' pain?

This will be your defining moment. Go back to the responses you wrote down in the box above. You will find that those you spoke to can express that defining moment and the difference it has made to their outlook and their career.

Being involved in research is one way that nurses can make a difference on a scale that is wider than the day-to-day care of their patients. However, nurse researchers do not need to work with patient care *or* research; they can, and they do, do both.

Being a researcher may not be on your priority list just now, but one day it may be. This is the way it is because you are intelligent enough to be doing one of the most demanding courses available. You are courageous enough to enter a profession that is well outside your comfort zone. You want to make things better for those who suffer. You are the stuff of progress, initiative and adventure. You could become a great researcher.

In the coming years you will be stamping your own mark on nursing and re-fashioning it to improve it and make it right for the years ahead. There can be no doubt that research will play a bigger part in nursing in the future, in your future. The migration of nursing to a research and evidence-led profession is already under way. In the years to come, there will be no confusion about what nursing research is or where it can be found; it will be everywhere. This shouldn't be frightening because you already value exactly what research values – that is, practice, a clear, objective focus and a demand that nursing should never rest on its laurels but should instead be constantly researching new ways to deliver better, more effective care.

This chapter started by wondering where research could be found, and we thought that research must be both academic and irrelevant to the practice of nursing. We have come to see that research will develop in the future as the profession of nursing develops. We have also seen that research is far from being dry and academic; rather, it is a practical endeavour, goaled to improve the care that nurses are able to deliver. Research in nursing is essential because nursing will never be content with what it knows and what it can do. Nursing will always strive to make things better.

Example from practice

What do you want to be doing in five years' time?

Just now you will be occupied with successfully completing your course. You will be looking forward to being a staff nurse. You may not have looked much further than this; after all, this is quite a big achievement. However, it can be useful to think about a longer-term vision. Take a few moments to jot down where you would like to be at the following points in your career:

- In two years' time, or when you first feel that you are expert at your first post-qualifying post in nursing.
- In five years' time, when you will have lots of experience and may want to branch out and specialise.
- When you have been in nursing long enough that people look to you because of your experience and knowledge.

What kind of nurse do you want to be?

Give this some thought and then tick just one of the following boxes:

- I want to be a proper nurse, to look like a nurse and be respected as a nurse. I want to be like the other nurses who work in my branch area and work as a member of a team, with them. ☐
- I want to work with other nurses and be good at what I do, but I also want to find my own mark and make my own unique contribution to nursing and patient care. ☐

Which one is correct? That depends on you; both represent a significant achievement. However, there is an important distinction between the two answers. It is worth some thought. Pester the researchers in your faculty just one more time and ask them which box they would tick.

Concluding remarks

It is often thought that research is a dry and academic subject and one that is not at all suited to the very practical orientation that nurses have to their work. However, this chapter has tried to show that this is far from being the case and that research and evidence-based practice are at the very heart of nursing and that not only is it easy to understand but that you already understand it and practise it. Research drives nursing to become ever better at delivering care to sick people. Research is not as clearly visible as is orthopaedics or surgery; this is because, rather than being a sub-discipline of nursing, research actually underpins everything that nurses do. In this way, to find research, one needs not to look around oneself but rather to look at the ground upon which practice is standing.

Summary

- It is easy to be blind to the nursing research happening around us, but examples of research affecting practice are everywhere; we only need to look.

- Nursing is a practice discipline. Its rightful orientation is the care of the patient. Nursing research has exactly the same orientation and is performed by nurses exercising the same orientation they had as students – that is, to improve patient care.

- Research is an eminently practical and focused activity.

- The principles of research are easy to understand. You are already familiar with research, and you practise it in your daily life as an intelligent student with great potential. This chapter has tried to persuade you to look at research in a new light, but it has not had to 'teach' you anything.

- Your goal at this point in your career is to become a skilled nurse, to be accepted by the health-care team and to have developed a sense of mastery over the clinical field in which you will choose to work. Your goal is entirely appropriate and creditable. However, there will come a time when you will want to exercise your professional duty to nursing as a whole, and to help nurses all over the world deliver better care. This is an orientation that you should begin to foster now. Being involved in research is one way in which you can make a difference on such a scale as this.

Further reading

Fessele, K. (2007). 'Behind the scenes of clinical research: from trial to triumph'. *ONS Connect* **22**(8): 8–12.

Smith, M. C. (2007). 'Nursing research: what is it and how can dermatology nurses use it?'. *Dermatology Nursing* **19**(5): 435–438.

Snow, T. (2008). 'Is nursing research catching up with other disciplines?'. *Nursing Standard* **22**(19): 12-13.

Winsett, R. P. and A. K. Cashion (2007). 'The nursing research process'. *Nephrology Nursing Journal* **34**(6): 635-643.

References

Austin, L. (1988). 'The salt bath myth'. *Nursing Times* **84**(9): 79.

Baskett, P. and D. Zideman (2005). 'European Resuscitation Guidelines'. *Resuscitation* **67**(Supplement 1): 1-190.

Canning, D., J. P. Rosenberg and P. Yates (2007). 'Therapeutic relationships in specialist palliative care nursing practice'. *International Journal of Palliative Nursing* **13**(5): 222-229.

Charters, A. (2000). 'Wound glue: a comparative study of tissue adhesives'. *Accident & Emergency Nursing* **8**(4): 223-227.

Helberg, D., E. Mertens, R. J. G. Halfens and T. Dassen (2006). 'Treatment of pressure ulcers: results of a study comparing evidence and practice'. *Ostomy Wound Management* **52**(8): 60.

Kieslich, C., G. Marquardt, G. Galow, R. Lorenz and G. Jacob (2001). 'Neurological and mental outcome after severe head injury in childhood: a long term follow-up of 318 children'. *Disability and Rehabilitation* **23**(15): 665-669.

Meyers, T. A., D. J. Eichhorn, C. E. Guzzetta, A. P. Clark, J. D. Klein and E. Taliaferro (2004). 'Family presence during invasive procedures and resuscitation: the experience of family members, nurses, and physicians ... reprinted with permission from the American Journal of Nursing, 2000;100(2):32-42'. *Topics in Emergency Medicine* **26**(1): 61-73.

Rognstad, M. and O. Aasland (2007). 'Change in career aspirations and job values from study time to working life'. *Journal of Nursing Management* **15**(4): 424-432.

Walsh, M. and P. Ford (1989). *Nursing Rituals, Research and Rational Actions*. London: Heinemann.

Wigert, H., R. Johansson, M. Berg and A. Hellström (2006). 'Mothers' experiences of having their newborn child in a neonatal intensive care unit'. *Scandinavian Journal of Caring Sciences* **20**(1): 35-41.

Windich-Biermeier, A., I. Sjoberg, J. C. Dale, D. Eshelman and C. E. Guzzetta (2007). 'Effects of distraction on pain, fear, and distress during venous port access and venipuncture in children and adolescents with cancer'. *Journal of Pediatric Oncology Nursing* **24**(1): 8-19.

Chapter 2
The literature: looking at what we already know

CHAPTER OBJECTIVES

The objectives for this chapter are to:

- Differentiate professional literature from other, less formal literature

- Recognise the rationale for using the professional literature in preference to other forms of writing

- Be able to locate the professional literature

- Begin to develop the confidence required to make sense of the professional literature, in part, by appreciating that the reader's skills in relation to their writing at this level are already well developed

- Appreciate the value of professional writing to the development of nursing

- Be determined to share ideas with others and so participate fully in professional life.

Chapter outline

Research is a very practical activity. However, you could be excused for thinking that research exists only as a great deal of written material, much of it both long and complex. This chapter aims to clarify the purpose of the professional and research literature and how it fits in with the ethos of professional nursing. This chapter will argue that although nursing does have a practice orientation, the professional and research literature is necessary for nursing to develop and to progress. This chapter will look at the differences between the professional and the research literature, how to find the literature and how to make sense of it.

Just a thought

Are you a typical student? It does not take long for students (and staff) to realise that the Internet can be a very useful tool. Answers to almost any question can be found easily using one of the freely available search engines. In fact, the search engine and the Internet itself have become such an integral part of the computer that it is hard to imagine the point of a computer without these facilities. So, it is not surprising that students today use their Internet search engine (e.g. Google) where, years ago, students would have used the university library. Indeed, it is probably the case that some students have yet to find their way to the library with its intimidating edifice, complicated catalogue and knowledgeable librarians. The university library can be an intimidating place.

It is common sense that directs students to what seems to be easily the best source of knowledge: the Internet search engine. However, from time to time, it may be better to turn your computer off for a while and go to your university library. Here's why:

There are some very special people found in a university library: other students. These students don't talk, they don't eat and they are never seen to drink beer. These students are studying; they are focusing their whole mind on one single activity. There is silence except for the sound of the occasional dusty volume being moved from shelf to table. There is an atmosphere here that is conducive to study. Here, in the library, there is a strange, if not decidedly odd, camaraderie of fellow students, though communication between student and student is limited to the occasional eye contact, grimace or smile. This is powerful stuff; not only do essays get written in double quick time but we have known life-long relationships be formed in the library, grown up from all that eye contact and from the grimaces and smiles indicative of a common understanding. So, be wary of the library: you may get your essay written ten times faster than if you used Google at home but you could end up with a friend to carry your essay home for you.

Research is just common sense. In this, it is no different from dealing with any other everyday challenge. It follows that science that is grounded in research is just common sense too. Research is about questioning, it is about those situations where we are not sure we have an answer. However, not everyone questions; you may know people whose lives are chiefly orientated to 'doing the right thing', to complying with the rules set by others and for whom wondering and working things out for themselves seem never to be part of their lives. So let us be clear: although research is simply common sense, it is not for everyone. To be involved in research, even to take it seriously, one needs to be prepared to wonder, to ask questions and to have the confidence in yourself sufficient to believe that you can make a difference.

It is perhaps too easy to think that there must be someone out there who knows the answer to a question or that there are others who will sort out a problem for us. Research is for those of us who are prepared to question, prepared to believe that our views and our intellectual skills are valuable and that we can and should use these skills to contribute to the common weal.[1]

It has already been made clear that you are not just anyone. In fact, you are a very special person. You are prepared to challenge yourself in studying nursing so that you can practise as a nurse and make a difference to people's lives. There are times in this process when you will simply absorb the knowledge that other people possess. However, nursing is not just a job; nurses have a professional orientation, which in part means that they accept an obligation to make a unique contribution to nursing. In other words, you are a wondering, questioning person. You are amazing. You already possess the confidence to know you can make a unique contribution to nursing. You respect those people with more experience and knowledge than yourself, but at the same time you believe you can contribute to the knowledge-base of nursing, improve it, make it better; importantly, you intend to do just that in the years to come.

It is important to understand the points made here, because in this chapter we will begin the search that is 're-search'. In doing this we will not ask ourselves why we should bother or why we can't simply ask a more experienced person to tell us the answer to our question.

Searching the existing literature is near the beginning of the research process. Here, we want to find out what has already been written on the subject. We want to understand what is already understood by others and what research has already been completed on the subject in question. In searching the literature,

---

[1] *Common weal* means for the good of everyone

however, we are not content to find out what that literature contains. Rather, we intend to use this knowledge to create more knowledge through research. We are motivated to do this for one very simple reason: we wish to contribute to that body of knowledge, to add to it through our own intelligence and endeavour. We are thus motivated because we are determined that, in our working life as a nurse, we will make a difference.

Why look at the existing literature?

Research is a significant investment. Most research projects cost money and take a considerable amount of time to complete. It is necessary to make sure that we do not waste our time by, for example, conducting a study that may already have been done by someone else.

There is more than one way of conducting a study. Research techniques, or methodologies, are developing all the time. It makes sense to look at how other people have conducted their studies in order to find out which methodologies are most successful in different circumstances.

Research is designed to do just one thing – that is, to build on the discipline's body of knowledge. This building should be cumulative and organised. If we were building a house, it would be no use building the ground floor before we had built the foundations, and so it is with research. So, we need to know what research has already been done, so that we can build on it in a logical (common-sense) and ordered manner.

It is sometimes necessary to find out what is *not* known and what has *not* been researched so far. Sometimes, people have a new idea and they wish to initiate a completely new line of enquiry. Even here, the researcher will need to search the literature in order to be sure that his or her idea really is new. It is in the nature of things that this is a relatively unusual position to be in. However, nursing has made use of qualitative research to explore new understandings of the experiences of patients and clients (Terry and Carroll 2008). In fact, nursing is quite good at using novel and flexible approaches in research. Nurses seem also to be good at focusing their research on the lived experiences of patients and clients and even other nurses (Chung *et al.* 2005). In these situations it is not uncommon for whole new lines of enquiries to be initiated. Even here, it is still important to be aware of what (if any) research has been completed on the subject in question and to be aware of the methodologies used to achieve both the collection and the analysis of data. All this requires a search of the existing literature to take place.

What is 'the literature'?

We need to recognise that there is a difference between the content of most webpages and what exists as the professional literature. Let us be clear about what it is that constitutes the professional literature.

Professional literature:

- is written using an accepted standard of language that is respectful of other professionals, even when criticising their work (Happell 2008);

- employs language that is non-emotional and is objective rather than subjective;

- is focused on the subject in question;

- contains both analysis and synthesis. The result is an objective and systematic exploration of the matter in question. Synthesis is to accept the challenge set by conflicting sets of information. It is never sufficient, for example, to write that one research project suggests one thing and another suggests something else – somehow, coherent sense needs to be made of the conflicting information;

- is made subject to peer review: no professional material is published without being judged by the author's peers. This peer review process is anonymous: the reviewers do not know the identity of the author and, in responding to the reviewers' comments, the author is not aware of the reviewers' identity. It is in this way that the written material is judged on its own merits and not on the past achievements or reputation of the author.

All professional literature complies with the criteria listed above. In confining our search to the professional literature, we rule out:

- many books, especially those that are aimed at telling us how to do things;

- most of the magazines you can find in a newsagent's shop;

- most webpages and most of the material that can be found by an Internet search engine.

However, finding the professional literature has never been easier, at least for university students with access to online databases.

At this point, we need to note that there are essentially two kinds of professional literature. The first is sometimes called 'anecdotal', which simply means that it is not research. This is not a lower class of literature; it is just that professionals and academics write about all manner of things and do not confine their work to research. This anecdotal literature complies fully with our criteria, but it isn't research. It follows that the second kind of professional literature is that based on research. Typically, when a research project is completed, the research team will publish the research, so that others can read it and be aware of the results of the study. It is important for us to be able to distinguish between anecdotal and research literature. Here, we are interested in research and the knowledge and evidence that research produces. We may use the anecdotal literature for ideas and for background reading, but most of our attention will be confined to the research literature.

It is easy to tell the difference between anecdotal and research literature. One is not research and one is research. However, students do sometimes confuse the two. A single journal may publish both kinds of material. Anecdotal literature can be, and often is, searching, critical and analytical, and it may consider existing research. Sometimes students confuse a published literature review with research because the authors have researched the topic. Real research, however, involves collecting new data or at least performing a new analysis on data.

Anecdotal literature is not less worthy than research literature. Anecdotal literature performs an essential role in professional life. However, it does represent a lower level of knowledge than does research. In practice, when we search the literature to inform a research project that we intend to undertake, we are interested mainly in the research literature – that is, what research has been done before, how it was done, how successful it was and what new information it produced.

Embedded in these criteria for professional and research literature are the foundations of science itself. These criteria are so important that they have created what we know of as 'science'. However, there is no rocket science here. What distinguishes professional literature and scientific literature (which is much the same thing) from other forms of writing are criteria that can be readily understood and that are common sense.

So, if this is science, what is art? In what way is the study of English literature, for example, different from scientific writing? The distinction between science and the academic study of art does seem quite unclear. Perhaps it is not for nothing that English literature and science can both be studied at university; they are both intellectual disciplines. Perhaps the distinction between the academic study of art and that of science does not really add up to much. So, perhaps the use of the term 'professional literature' rather than 'scientific literature' is appropriate. It is certainly the case that academics who write professionally about Dickens's books, for example, will employ all of the criteria listed above. Perhaps science itself is something of a fabrication; certainly, there seems to be confusion about what exactly it is. However, what is important here is that we are clear about the meaning of the term 'research'. Both the arts and the sciences conduct research, and the criteria they use for what they write is the same. This point is salient to nursing. Nurses do often find that they are more interested in the softer side of science. It is not surprising that nurses are often interested in human experience, of pain, grief, psychiatric illness, parenting, illness and a thousand other interesting topics. We can perhaps now see that the distinction between art and science is not very useful.

Even if we were clear about what constitutes science, we could still not say that nursing is a science. Like medicine, nursing is a practice discipline, and the word 'practitioner' seems to suit nursing better than the word 'scientist'. Nursing is a field of practice, it is not a science. However, science can be and often is found in nursing. Nursing becomes scientific whenever a professional nurse seeks to address a topic using the criteria of respect for other professionals, objectivity, focus, and the collection and analysis of new data, and when that nurse seeks to publish his or her work by subjecting it to peer review.

So, perhaps we can begin to see the value of the professional literature. The professional literature is not just writing or published stuff. Actually, it has a value commensurate with the adoption of the criteria identified above. The adoption of these criteria sets professional literature aside from, if not above, much of everything else that is written. Much that is written in books and on webpages is both good and useful, but the professional literature is different. Furthermore, the research literature represents what is science in each discipline; in medicine, nursing, English literature and the history of art.

How do I trust the literature?

In practice, there is a hierarchy of quality in the nursing literature. Books are usually at the bottom of the hierarchy because they tend to limit their content to description. In practice, there is very little research to be found in books. The research that does exist in books is usually limited to brief description of what research is available. This can come as a surprise to the new student because those outside professional life often consider books to be clever things. Maybe they are clever, but sadly very little research is found in books and so books seldom meet our purpose. Books are useful when it comes to describing things, such as when you are learning how to practise surgical nursing. However, for evidence of real research, we almost always have to look to journals and to a subset of journals that are regarded as academic.

It is not uncommon for the whole notion of research to be dismissed by under-graduate students. After all, you will be aware of conflicting research. One study tells us one thing, and another study tells us something that conflicts with the first study. It is not unnatural to see this as evidence that research is untrustworthy. Let us look at the argument that research is valueless because of the way that one study so often disagrees with another study. Well, it's true: studies do often find evidence that contradicts earlier studies.

Research is not an infallible endeavour. Researchers are human beings; they may be clever (just like you) but they are not perfect (just like you). Researchers don't always get everything right. More usually, however, researchers do manage to do the best they can with the resources available to them. It is just that some things are very difficult to research. Researchers usually do their best in such circum-stances, but sometimes the circumstances defeat them.

Example from practice

Family-centred care has been a defining concept in paediatric nursing for at least the past 30 years. It is a mode of nursing that emphasises the status of the child patient as a member of a family and the role the family should always have in the delivery of medical and nursing care. The approach to nursing also emphasises the child's psychological, devlopmental and social needs and the way that these are intimately related to the functioning of the family within which the child plays a central part. Shields *et al.* (2007) undertook a systematic review* of family-centred care in order to determine what evidence existed to support its continuing practice. However, the authors of the systematic review found that there were no existing studies of a suitable quality. Family-centred care is practised by most, perhaps all, paediatric nurses, and so it seems strange that no good-quality research exists on the matter. However, family-centred care is a collective term for a wide range of approaches to care, some of which are conceptual rather than practical. Paediatric nurses work with a large number of children, from babies to young adults, and a wide range of illnesses. In this way, family-centred care is prob-ably un-researchable. Rather, it is necessary to research each individual aspect of family-centred care. Fortunately, evidence of this kind does exist. For example, Kain *et al.* (2007) found that the application of the principles of family-centred care did help children who were waiting for surgery. Nevertheless, the work by Shields *et al.* (2007) does illustrate the way in which some research may simply be impossible and (by implication) a lot of research maybe very difficult to do well.

* A systematic review is a collection of the best research on a particular topic where an attempt is made to pool the data from all the studies and to analyse the new, larger pool of data. In this context, the word 'meta-analysis' is sometimes used.

Research should be, and usually is, a cumulative endeavour. One research project builds upon another. It is not at all unnatural that, at one point in time, the available research appears to be contradictory. In the fullness of time, we are able to see that the research was progressing towards a known goal. When that goal is achieved, the progress can be seen in perspective and it can be seen that the research was pushing forward the front line of knowledge. With each push, however, there often comes a backlash of evidence as areas of knowledge defend the onslaught. Perhaps it is like a battle. There are winners and losers and there are reputations at stake. Researchers are human and they will, and indeed they should, try to defend their position against the advance of new knowledge. New research, producing new knowledge, should not have it easy. Such new knowledge should be challenged and challenged again until there is nothing left to challenge, until we can be certain that the new knowledge is right, correct, certain and that it should therefore replace the old knowledge. The point is that there is friction and challenge here, which does release energy. We should expect this and welcome it. For such friction is part of the advancement of new knowledge. Nothing else would be right; new knowledge should be challenged and then it should be challenged again. We must be sure that what we know is correct and that it should rightfully replace the knowledge that has gone before.

So, we are not going to be put off by conflicting research and disagreement. However, there is such a thing as poor-quality research. It is often difficult for the student to judge what is good or not-so-good research. After all, most students have little or no experience of actually doing any research. To expect students to judge the quality of research is like asking them to judge the performance of a neurosurgeon or a deep-sea diver. Until one has gained experience of doing a job, one is not in a very good position to judge it. What makes this matter worse is that the research literature can be very difficult to understand, and inexperienced students will often deal with this by confining their search to the less academic (popular) journals. The inevitable consequence of this is that they stumble across the less good research literature. It can be better to confine the search to the more academic journals. While this can yield up research papers that can be difficult to understand, at least one can be assured that the quality of the research is better than poor. The message is clear: don't shy away from the more academic, less popular journals. Rather, try to read them, and then read them again until they begin to make sense. This is not easy but it is better to grasp the nettle rather than settle for less.

Most online databases such as Academic Search Elite (EBSCO Host: **http://search.ebscohost.com**) will enable you to tick a box next to your search term to indicate that you are only interested in peer-reviewed articles (always tick this box, as in Figure 2.1). This all you need to do. However, it is also possible to

Scholarly (Peer Reviewed) Journals ☑

Figure 2.1 Ticking the box indicates that you're interested only in peer-reviewed journals
Source: © EBSCO Publishing, Inc., 2009. All rights reserved.

choose only those journals with an impact factor. The impact factor measures the number of times that articles in a particular journal are cited – that is, referenced within other publications. In this way, the impact factor is a measure of how used are the articles published within a particular journal. So, the impact factor is a measure of the quality of the journal, not the individual papers published by that journal. If you wish to take this route, you can decide to confine yourself to journals that have an impact factor or you can look at those journals with the highest impact factor. It can be useful to know which journals have the highest impact factor but, other than that, the baseline of peer-reviewed journal is sufficient[2].

Where do I find the professional literature?

Most people are used to using the Internet and are adept at using search engines such as Google® to find information. Google can be used to find information about almost anything, and it is a great resource. However, it isn't a good idea to use Google to search for literature, as there are better ways of doing this. Instead of using Google, try the variety of online databases that are purchased by your university and that are available on the Internet (online) and are usually accessed via university library webpages.

If you are a university student, you will have easy access to these electronic journals and to online databases that do a great job of tracking down the material you are looking for. Things are much more difficult if you do not have this free access to the online journals. It is probably not enough to subscribe to just one journal. Today, there are so many journals that one journal cannot hope to publish all the best research articles. If you are not a university student, then it may be best to pay a subscription to just one of the online databases (there is a list at the end of this chapter). This will make available to you a whole raft of journals. Librarians have been particularly adept at keeping up to date with the changing style of library usage. Today, the average librarian possesses a wealth of knowledge about which online journals are available and which ones are best for which purposes. The average librarian has become an expert in the use of computers to access

[2] If you want to know more about impact factors, find the *Journal of Citation Reports* on your university library webpage.

good-quality material via online databases and online journals. So the message is clear: use your librarian. This often involves meekly entering the ivory tower of the library, searching out a busy-looking librarian and admitting to being lost. Don't worry, we have all been there.

Now, the impatient librarian does exist. Today, the average librarian has degrees to spare. However, where a little respect is shown, the librarian will be keen to whisk the average student off his or her feet and wrap that poor student in arms of benevolent guidance. Being a student (and we never stop being one of those) is an exercise in resource management. Most students don't have much in the way of resources, and so the good use of what resources are available is much required. The librarian is the student's best birthday present, a free, knowledgeable and willing resource, a positive fountain of knowledge, there just to serve you. Use your librarian.

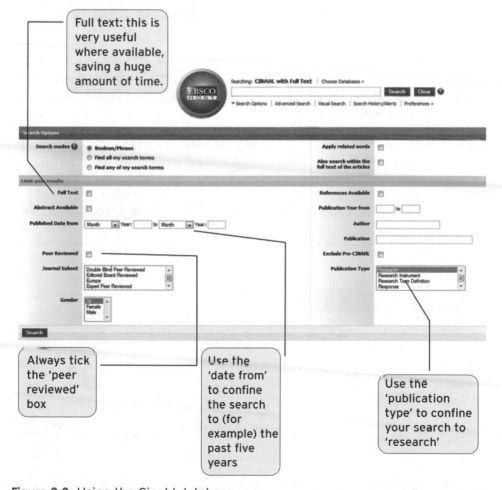

Figure 2.2 Using the Cinahl database
Source: © EBSCO Publishing, Inc., 2009. All rights reserved.

An example of a suitable online database is Cinahl (EBSCO Host: **http://search.ebscohost.com**). Using such a database is very easy. Simply enter your search string (e.g. 'pain AND child') into the search box and then (Figure 2.2 on p. 35):

- always tick the 'peer reviewed' box;

- select the 'publication type' to 'research'; options to search for particular types of research such as double-blind control trials, may also be available;

- select the 'full text' option to save you much time in finding and ordering articles via your library;

- confine the date of publication to (for example) the past five years. This can be useful if you want the most up-to-date research and if leaving the option unticked results in too many articles being found.

Figure 2.3 shows the first few results from our search for research on 'child AND pain'.

So, searching for and finding published research is easy. Increasingly, the databases to which university students have access contain the downloadable electronic version of published material. There is no good reason for failing to use these online databases.

Search engines such as Google do not tend to find the professional literature. They may find secondary references, but it will be more profitable to use one

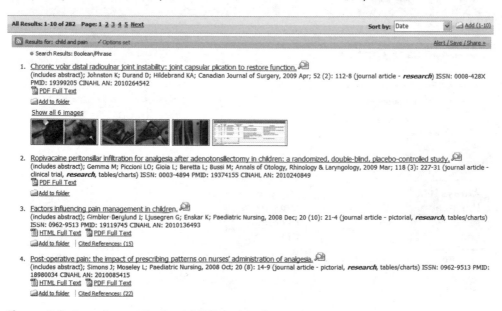

Figure 2.3 Search results for 'child' and 'pain'
Source: © EBSCO Publishing, Inc., 2009. All rights reserved.

of the Web-based databases that are specifically designed to hold professional literature. As a student of a UK university (and most non-UK universities), you will not have to pay to use these databases. It takes no more than half an hour to become relatively proficient at using these databases. So, while the rest of the world is happily using Google, you should be surfing elsewhere.

In the past few years, another useful source of published research has become available: the Cochrane Library (**http://www3.interscience.wiley.com**) is essentially another online resource, but it focuses on systematic reviews and controlled trials (Greenhalgh 1997). Controlled trials can be found elsewhere (although the Cochrane Library is an excellence source), but the Cochrane Library is the best place to go for systematic reviews.

New words

Systematic review A relatively new form of research that collects together all the best research on a particular topic and attempts to make sense of the resulting collection of studies (Greenhalgh 1997). Often, a systematic review will pool the data from several studies and run an analysis, known as a 'meta-analysis', on the pooled data. Where successful, this effectively increases the sample size and can offer up new information that was not available by looking at each individual study. As such, a systematic review can constitute new research. Full access to the Cochrane Library will be available via your university library webpage.

Randomised control trial (RCT) An experiment or prospective research study that has at least one control group and where randomisation is used to control bias. Blinding is also used in RCTs; this is where the participant and perhaps the researcher, are not aware of which research group the participant has been allocated to. Blinding helps to reduce the risk of bias. The RCT tries to mimic the archetypal laboratory experiment by controlling any variable that might impact on the research.

The Cochrane Library is becoming the single best source for research literature. However, it tends only to hold good-quality quantitative studies. It may be necessary to look elsewhere for more explorative or qualitative work.

For the student who is starting out on their journey into the research literature, the sources Cinahl and the Cochrane Library should prove sufficient. Between them you can find hundreds of thousands of research papers.

Making sense of published research

Research is easy to understand. Although it often looks complex, underneath all the apparent gobbledegook is something essentially very simple. So, when you look at your first research paper, you could be forgiven for thinking that this claim has been overstated. It is true that research does often look very complex. This is due in part to the language used by researchers and in part to the huge variety of research methods in use. Nursing students are often more bewildered by research than are students of other disciplines such as medicine. Nursing is not a pure discipline, such as psychology or geography; rather, it is eclectic and diverse. Because of this, nursing employs a huge range of research methodologies, embracing as it does both the qualitative and the quantitative paradigms.

New words

Qualitative Essentially, explorative research that deals with words rather than numbers.

Quantitative Essentially, research that deals with numbers.

Perhaps you could get help by taking your research paper to your friendly university lecturer so that he or she can explain it all to you in simple English. This is a good idea, but it can be difficult to pin down a lecturer. Lecturers are very busy people – busy trying to hide from students holding long and complicated research papers. However, it is a good idea to try, so take your research paper and seek out your lecturer. Insist on it, don't accept any excuses, don't take any prisoners. Part of the problem here is that a complicated research paper can make the average student feel inadequate, perhaps even stupid. The danger, of course, is that our student will achieve a tutorial, only to fail to understand anything the lecturer said and only to feel even more stupid than was the case before. None of us likes to admit that we can't understand a word of what is written in front of us.

Take your research paper to a nice quiet place such as a library and try to understand it. It might not be easy. You will probably need a dictionary to look up all the new words – but do it all the same. Don't worry if it takes you all day or all week – it will *not* mean that you are stupid. There is a learning curve here: you have to climb the steep edifice of that curve before it begins to flatten out a little. If you expect the task to be difficult, then you will not feel quite so threatened when it proves to be difficult.

You may need to read the paper several times, but eventually you will make progress and it will become a little more clear. Now take it to your lecturer. Whatever excuse you gave yourself for not doing so is just that: an excuse to protect your self-confidence. Understand that this will take courage – but do it all the same. Go with a list (written down) of things that you do understand about the paper and a list of things you don't understand. Tell your lecturer what you think you understand about the paper and then the things you don't understand.

The point here is that it is easy to feel overwhelmed by the apparent complexity of the average research paper. This is a normal reaction. It does not prove that you are stupid; it proves only that you are human. Treat the paper like an invading army of Martians, something to be both attacked and defeated. Have courage, know that your mind is as keen as anyone else's, be prepared for a struggle and for set-backs, but be determined to conquer that research paper. By the end of this process the research paper will be lying exhausted at your feet, begging for mercy. It will be defeated, its complicated language will have been translated into plain English, its methodology will be exposed as nothing more than a common-sense way of finding an answer to the question at hand, and the analysis, that array of frightening numbers and words, will be seen for what it is – the result of a clear and logical exploration of the data.

The chapters following this one will guide you through the process of making sense of research papers. For now:

- don't be scared;

- make sure that you are looking at a research paper. The paper should contain an analysis of data. The data may be numbers (quantitative) or words (qualitative), but there should be new information there, derived from a data collection. Don't confuse research with a literature review, even where this reviews previous research;

- try not to use secondary papers (reports of other people's research);

- you will be used to critiquing things; however, try to go beyond criticising the researchers for what you think they have got wrong, because:

  - the people who published the research know more about it than you are likely to do; in criticising them, you may simply be exposing your own lack of understanding;
  - the main reason for research being imperfect is that some things are just very difficult to research. It is often impossible to use the most robust methodologies. For example, qualitative research is sometimes criticised for not coming close to the standards for a double-blind controlled trial, as used

in most medical drug research. However, there are times when only the explo-rative nature of qualitative research will yield up the information that is being sought. Students new to research often fail to understand the real-world diffi-culties and constraints of research. People new to research often criticise researchers for failing to do what is, in fact, impossible. Such criticism is likely to do nothing more than expose the student's lack of understanding;

- be sure that you report what the study found – that is, the results and not just the methodology (how the study was done). Make sure that you under-stand the results. If you are not sure how to interpret the results, read the paper again and then read it again, looking up all the words and phrases with which you are unfamiliar. If you still don't understand the results, ask your lecturer to interpret them for you;

- make sure that you comment on the implications (as you see them) of the study. There will be implications for further study and for nursing.

It is easy to be too descriptive when reviewing a research paper. You need to go beyond summarising it. Your report should have your ideas in it. There will need to be some description in your work, but there should also be an account of your ideas. Your section on the implications of the study is an excellent place in which to document some of your own ideas, your own thoughts and your own arguments.

Another thought – why do students write so many essays?

Let us understand this – students do not write essays so that they can be tested on the amount and depth of their knowledge. There are better ways of testing knowledge and it would be unforgivable to cause so many hours of work and the use of so many trees (paper) just to test students' knowledge and understanding. If we wanted only to test students' knowledge and understand-ing, we could simply talk to them, as in a viva, or give them a written examination with short-answer questions. Just think of the time and paper that would save. No, the rationale for the use of essays lies elsewhere.

An essay is an exercise in professional communication. An essay is the stu-dent's version of a published paper. It is about the same length as a published paper and it has the same characteristics as a published paper. These charac-teristics are that the essay:

- is written using an accepted standard of language;

- uses a discussion and arguments that are non-emotional and objective rather than subjective;

- is focused on the subject in question;

- 'tells a story': it contains a thesis – that is, a logical and integrated set of ideas that have a purpose, perhaps to inform the reader of something new or to enable the reader to see something in a new light. In achieving this, there is evidence of analysis and of the synthesis of existing and new ideas. In this way, the essay is a communication that goes way beyond summarising what already exists in other people's work. The essay is all about the student's own ideas;

- is made subject to assessment.

You have seen this list before, in the criteria for professional literature. So it is that in writing essays the student learns about writing professionally. Communication (sometimes in writing) is a requirement of professional life. Writing professionally is a vital component of both practice and research. The professional nurse has a duty, not only to his or her patients for today but for nursing, the state of the discipline of nursing and its progress. In this, the nurse is responsible not only for the job undertaken today but also for the nursing that other nurses are able to do, today and in the future. The nurse has a responsibility to make nursing better, to improve it, so that tomorrow other nurses can do the job better than we can do it today.

So it is that the nurse has a duty not only to improve his or her patient care but to do that and then to tell every other nurse, so that their care can be improved too. There would be no point in improving practice or in conducting research if we then kept this new information hidden from others. We have a duty to publish our efforts, so that others can examine them, judge their worth and, where appropriate, incorporate the new knowledge into their own research and their own practice.

So there is a purpose in writing essays. You will have written so many of them that by the end of your course you will be good at it. That is how it should be.

You will learn to practise nursing competently. However, this is not enough. You are nursing's future and you have a role to play in making nursing better. As part of this, you will have to tell others about your achievements – and you will be glad that you learned how to write a good essay – and the rest of the profession will be glad too.

Concluding remarks

The research and professional literature exists as an essential part of nursing and of research. Not everyone likes to spend all their time reading. So, it is important to be able to search for the best literature quickly and to discern the salient points from that literature in a focused and efficient manner. In practice, the literature is the way in which both nurses and researchers communicate their work to others. From the literature, we can see what is already known. Being informed of what is already known, we can begin the process of moving that knowledge-base forward. No professional can be satisfied with the way things are; all professionals have ideas about how to make things better. The literature is the starting block for those ideas to be tested by research and for them to lead to new insights and new practices in patient care.

Summary

- The professional literature is different from less formal literature. Professional literature is written and published to a standard, where principally it is objective and made subject to peer review.

- The professional literature is not best accessed via Internet search engines, but rather exists in Web-based databases such as that provided by Cinahl. It can also be found in university libraries where much expertise exists to help both the new student and the seasoned researcher to find information.

- The professional literature helps to define a profession. It is important because it is the main way in which nurses communicate their work and their research.

- The professional literature can be hard to understand. However, you are not only well on the way to being able to understand it and use it effectively; you are also advantaged in that you are pretty good at creating professional literature. The essays you have been asked to write during your course of study are the beginning of your publishing career. If you can write an essay, then you can write a paper and seek to get that paper submitted for publication.

- It is not enough to learn nursing. No profession can survive on what people already know. It is necessary to make things better. You will want to have an active role in seeking out new knowledge. Having done that, you will want to tell everyone what you have found. Others will read what you have written because they will want to build on what you have achieved. They will look at the professional literature to find your work, and the result will be a nursing profession that is always looking forward and always trying to improve what it can do for the people it tries to help.

Further reading

An example of the way in which the professional literature is used to define the current state of nursing as a discipline:

Weaver, K. (2007). 'Ethical sensitivity: state of knowledge and needs for further research'. Nursing Ethics **14**(2): 141-155.

This article considers the extent to which one branch of nursing (maternal and child health) is orientated to research:

Oermann, M. H., D. A. Blair, K. Kowalewski, N. A. Wilmes and C. K. Nordstrom (2007). 'Citation analysis of the maternal/child nursing literature'. *Pediatric Nursing* **33**(5): 387.

Current attitudes to research (in this case, among psychiatric nurses):

Parahoo, K. (1999). 'Research utilization and attitudes towards research among psychiatric nurses in Northern Ireland'. *Journal of Psychiatric and Mental Health Nursing* **6**(2): 125-135.

Note that it is usually best to access the following websites via your university library webpage. If you try to access these sites from your home computer, you may find that you are denied access or are asked for payment. In practice, you will probably find that you have free access from your university computers and that your university computer centre staff will be able to tell you how to get the same free access from your home computer.

Ebscohost (for Cinahl and Academic Search Elite):

http://search.ebscohost.com/Community.aspx

The National Library for Health offers free access to the Cochrane Database (for systematic reviews and experimental research). The site also offers access to other databases that are normally paid-for resources:

http://www.library.nhs.uk/

References

Chung, B. P. M., T. K. S. Wong, E. S. B. Suen and J. W. Y. Chung (2005). 'SARS: caring for patients in Hong Kong'. *Journal of Clinical Nursing* **14**(4): 510–517.

Greenhalgh, T. (1997). 'How to read a paper: papers that summarise other papers (systematic reviews and meta-analyses)'. *British Medical Journal* **315**(7109): 672–675.

Happell, B. (2008). 'The responsibility of review: guidelines to promote professional courtesy and commitment through the peer review process'. *International Journal of Psychiatric Nursing Research* **13**(3): 1–9.

Kain, Z. N., A. A. Caldwell-Andrews, L. C. Mayes, M. E. Weinberg, S. M. Wang, J. E. MacLaren and R. L. Blount (2007). 'Family-centered preparation for surgery improves perioperative outcomes in children: a randomized controlled trial'. *Anesthesiology* **106**(1): 65–74.

Shields, L., J. Pratt, L. Davis and J. Hunter (2007). 'Family centred care for children in hospital'. *Cochrane Database of Systematic Reviews*(1): CD004811.

Terry, L. M. and J. Carroll (2008). 'Dealing with death: first encounters for first-year nursing students'. *British Journal of Nursing* **17**(12): 760–765.

Chapter 3
Evidence-based practice

Chapter outline

Having identified the meaning of research in the previous chapter, we look now at the related concept of evidence-based practice. We will see that although research may provide the best form of evidence (the best form of knowledge), there are other forms of evidence that are often used to support practice. This chapter will also look at some of the ways in which people sometimes avoid using evidence. The acquisition of evidence, through research or other means, must be carried out within the established principles of ethical conduct. This chapter will look at what this means for the researcher and for you, as you begin to make sense of nursing as an ethical and evidenced-based profession.

What is evidence-based practice?

Put simply, the term 'evidence-based practice' needs no interpretation: it is what it says it is – that is, practice based on evidence. However, there are two ways in which the term 'evidence-based practice' can be understood.

Meaning 1: the use of research as just one of many forms of evidence

It is possible to argue that there exists more than one form of evidence, with research being only one form or source of evidence. Research is arguably the best form of evidence, but there are reasons for the lack of availability of research in nursing:

- Research is expensive. In Britain, there are no well-defined funding streams for research in nursing. Good-quality research usually involves the employment of research assistants, and this is usually very expensive.

- It is not always possible to conduct research to a recognisable standard. Nursing functions with people, and in some situations research with people would place them at risk or would infringe their human rights. Research with babies, for example, is problematic because it is not possible to gain the informed consent of the babies themselves and because responsible adults are limited in the degree to which they can consent for children where the research may not be in their child's interest. So, research is sometimes difficult or impossible to do, and good research that meets the accepted standard for control and randomisation is very often impossible to conduct within the arena in which nurses operate.

In some ways, the use of alternative forms of evidence is justified. Where research conducted to scientific standards of control and randomisation is impossible to conduct, we have little alternative but to accept the use of research that does not meet these standards. In the same way, if research in any form is impossible, then there is little alternative but to accept other forms of evidence. Clearly, however, we need to insist on research evidence when such research is both possible and desirable, and we need to fully appreciate the dangers inherent in accepting forms of evidence that may be prone to error and that may be misleading.

The use of the term 'evidence-based practice' relates to an acceptance that forms of evidence other than that generated by research can be used appropriately. There is no universal agreement on such use of non-research evidence.

However, health care is replete with examples of practice based on non-research evidence, and so it is important to give this area some thought, if only with a couple of caveats:

- Where research conducted to scientific standards remains achievable, other forms of evidence should always be seen as less than adequate.

- Non-research evidence should be understood to be particularly vulnerable to flaw and error and to possess a capacity to mislead.

In short, research evidence is almost always the best form of evidence, and nursing should always seek evidence from research. However, other forms of evidence cannot be easily dismissed, may at the very least be interesting, and may all too often present the best evidence available to us at the moment.

Meaning 2: a process by which poor or ineffective practices are weeded out and better practice is identified and implemented

The term 'evidence-based practice' is also used to denote practice that is based on some form of evidence, as opposed to practice that fails to be supported by any form of evidence. The term 'evidence-based practice' was probably first used in medicine and reflected an attempt to weed out practices that had a basis only in tradition and experience or to ensure that such practices were properly evaluated and made subject to peer review.

It was perhaps the early use of the term 'evidence-based medicine' that encouraged the use of non-research forms of evidence. This was not because these forms of evidence were in any way considered superior to research but that *any* form of evidence was an evolutionary move in the right direction. Just to get medical practitioners to think about their practices and to look at what other practitioners were doing was a major and very important step forward for medicine. In other words, we need to see evidence-based practice in evolutionary terms. Medicine and nursing are evolving, trying to improve. Both disciplines have had to learn to stand before they could learn to walk, to look at their practice objectively before being able to subject it to research.

Non-research forms of evidence

Let's look at what other forms of evidence are sometimes used to support practice:

Peer review

Peer review is a central component of professional life and an important mechanism for ensuring that practice is supported by at least some form of evidence. Peer review can be applied to a new idea, a practice innovation, continuing professional registration, publication and just about every aspect of professional life.

A peer is someone like you, your equal. In this way, peer review for students would be undertaken by other students and not by academic or practice staff. Peer review for publication would be undertaken by people who are themselves nurses who publish their own work from time to time. Peer review in clinical practice is undertaken by other practitioners and not by managers or (usually) people from other professions.

Clinical audit

Clinical audit is, arguably, a form of research. However, it tends to be concerned with the collection of descriptive (as opposed to experimental) data, which have to do with documented standards of patient care. Audits do not usually achieve the standard of scientific research because they lack the necessary control of variables, and randomisation is seldom possible. Despite these failings, audits are used widely and do provide valuable feedback on measures of the quality of patient care.

Benchmarking

Benchmarking is a form of standard that is set by a community of practitioners, often by a local group of hospitals. A standard, or benchmark, is set and work takes place to establish that standard and perhaps to exceed it. The power of benchmarking lies within the liaison that takes place within the community of practitioners. In the case of a local group of hospital staff, this

community of practitioners might not have come together except for the purpose of establishing the benchmarking. So, benchmarking encourages liaison
outside one's own workplace; it has the effect of first equalising the standard
of care being practised in individual departments across a region or area and
then improving that standard further. Benchmarking is a mix of both peer
review and the development of standards. It has the advantage that the benchmark is set by practitioners rather than managers. In this way, the
development or initiative is fully owned by the practitioners themselves.

Established clinical expertise

Health-care practice is full of expert knowledge. Much of this knowledge has been
acquired through experience. However, experience is best used when it is shared
with others, debated in public and published. This offers the opportunity for other
experts to point out possible flaws in relation to the practice in question.

Although clinical expertise falls short of what research is able to offer, it should be
recognised that people know a lot of things that have never been subject to
research. Clinical expertise is a valuable resource. However, knowledge can sometimes be more subjective than objective, and it is possible for lots of very capable
people to believe that something is true when in fact it is not. There is a tendency
for us to think that something must be right if everyone believes it, but it is possible for everyone to be wrong. For this reason, it is important that clinical expertise
is made subject to close scrutiny and that it is evaluated objectively.

During much of the twentieth century, nurses did not allow parents to stay in
hospital with their sick children (Figure 3.1). Sometimes, parents were not even
allowed to visit their children, even when children were hospitalised for many
weeks and when they were seriously ill (Jolley 2007, 2008; Jolley and Shields
2009). It was thought by almost everyone, nurses, doctors and hospital admin-
istrators, that having parents in hospital with their children would cause the
sick child harm (see Duncombe 1979). Only after the Second World War did
people gradually come to appreciate that children had an important emotional
bond with their parents and that having parents stay with children in hospital
helped children considerably. So, just about everybody was wrong.

Figure 3.1 For most of the twentieth century, hospitalised children had to cope without their parents

Tradition

'We always do it this way.' Perhaps you have been frustrated by a senior nurse's desire to stick to the way things have always been done. Nurses should be open to new ideas but so too do they need to recognise the wisdom of the past. If a particular type of wound has been dressed in a particular way for the past 50 years, then maybe there is good reason for continuing this practice. We may not have good evidence to support the practice in question, but neither may we have good evidence to abandon the practice. We have already noted that lots of people can be uniformly incorrect. Nevertheless, the more people who support a particular approach to care, the more likely it is that they are right. It is the case that they could all be wrong and it is definitely the case that global assumptions for good practice should be questioned and objective data sought. Nevertheless, tradition should not be dismissed too readily. Practices do not become tradition overnight and, although the process that selects them may be less than scientific and less than rigorous, processes designed to identify flaws almost always exist in these cases. It follows that traditional techniques have stood the test of time and do therefore deserve to be taken seriously. This notwithstanding, every practitioner (including you and me) has the right to challenge tradition. Tradition is fairly low down the hierarchy of knowledge and as such it should expect to be challenged, even by the most junior of staff.

Experience

Experience is a little like tradition, except that it applies to only one individual. We should be careful before belittling experiences, and yet it is a long way from the evidence produced by research. We have probably all come across situations where patients are treated differently, even on the same ward, because two consultants have been trained using two different techniques. It takes little thought to appreciate the need here to evaluate the two procedures, for one is likely to be superior to the other.

Example from the literature and research

Western medicine is based on the principles of science and evidence-based practice. However, there are many parts of the world where western medicine has yet to develop or where it is in competition with traditional healing. The lack of evidence-based practice and research in traditional healing is often a cause for concern. However, the lack of evidence to support a particular practice does in no way mean that the practice is of poor quality. A lack of evidence simply means that we don't know whether something works. It follows that traditional practices should not be too readily dismissed. Xu *et al*. (2006) studied the practice of traditional healers in China who provide therapy for people with cancer. Their qualitative study found that patients did recieve some benefit from the traditional healers. Indeed, the researchers suggest that this particular model of cancer care should be evaluated more fully in order to determine whether it could be of benefit as an adjunct to western medicine.

Experience is more credible if it is supported by others and especially if it is formally critiqued by peer review, as when someone attempts to publish an article promoting a particular practice. Publishing is important because the process of getting a paper published opens it to peer review (all the articles in the professional press are peer-reviewed before being published). Once the paper is published, it can be read and critiqued by a large number of practitioners. Publishing ideas on an example of practice both tells other people about those ideas and exposes the ideas to critique. In this way, publishing is an important mechanism of ensuring that practice is evidence-based and is an essential element of professional life. We should all publish because we should all have ideas about how practice can be improved.

Example from the literature and research

Stewart (2006) describes the development of new guidelines for catheterisation at a particular hospital. This paper describes the challenges that were overcome when peer review was used to ensure that the new guidelines were properly evidence-based and accepted by both the medical and nursing staff. The author illustrates how practitioners can themselves take ownership of a new initiative and can work together successfully to achieve a change in practice and to ensure that practice continues to be based on the best available evidence.

Policy and guidelines

Government develops health policy, and hospitals develop clinical standards of one sort or another. Mechanisms are often put in place to maintain practice within the parameters of the policy in question. In most cases, the policies are reviewed and audited to ensure that they continue to be appropriate and effective. Policies and the effectiveness of them can be compared between health institutions, even to the point where league tables can be formulated so that people can see which health organisations are performing best. These league tables are based on data, but these data often fall short of scientific standards. Even so, these data can be considered to be a form of evidence. An example of this form of evidence is the government's criteria for waiting times in accident and emergency departments. In this case, the government established a policy that hospitals should work to reduce waiting times. Accident departments were then audited to provide data on waiting times and the improvement or otherwise of waiting times. Using these data, it is possible to compare one accident department with other accident departments.

Policy formation can sometimes be politically charged. Clearly, the policies themselves relate to the prevailing political will (to reduce accident department waiting times). This is usually sufficiently transparent. However, the collection of data can also be politically motivated, largely because it is related so closely to the interests of agencies such as government and National Health Service (NHS) trusts (see Castledine 2008). It follows that care needs to be taken to ensure that bias has not influenced the data or their analysis. It might be possible, for example, to record patients as having been discharged from the accident department even though it is known that they have not yet been admitted to a ward or been taken home. Formal research can also suffer from bias. However, mechanisms are set in place to ensure that bias is properly controlled. Clinical audit and the evaluation of policy decisions often fail to implement these controls. In any case, it is always necessary to be wary of any data, the collection of which may be politically motivated or may serve the interests of a person or agency.

Research that does not meet the standard of scientific criteria

Many studies are published that use methodologies that are inexpensive to implement but that fail to provide the best forms of control and randomisation. Such studies may suffer from the effect of bias or from the effect of one or more variables that have not been properly accounted for. It is debatable whether these studies add much to our knowledge and evidence base. However, it is probably appropriate to consider them here as providing a form of evidence outside the parameter of fully fledged research projects.

Dyer (1997) considers the relatively high proportion of small-scale and poorly controlled studies in the nursing literature. However, rather than criticising these less than perfect studies, Dyer takes the view that they are part of the evolution of research in nursing and that they should be considered a legitimate source of evidence upon which practice can be supported.

Practice that is supported by anecdotal evidence and by the literature

Anecdotal evidence means non-research evidence. We have seen that the professional literature can usefully be divided into two categories, research and anecdotal. In common usage, anecdotal means unreliable or subjective; however, it really has neither of these qualities – it is just *not* research. A typical example of anecdotal literature is a nursing care study in which the author discusses the care given to a particular patient. The purpose of the study might be to tell the reader about a nursing initiative or to inform less experienced nurses about the care in this case and the implications that care had for one patient.

It should be clear that there is nothing at all wrong with anecdotal literature; in fact, much of the nursing literature is anecdotal and it serves a very good purpose. Indeed, the anecdotal literature can be seen as the backbone of professional life. It is here that practitioners write about their initiatives so that others can learn from them and so for the express purpose of these initiatives being made open to critique by others. This is not research, but the combined effort of the original paper and the opportunity the rest of the profession has to critique that paper is as much evidence as anything else discussed here.

Example from the literature and research

Fiona Murphy (2006) published a care study in which she illustrated the use of a form of nursing assessment (Gordon's (1994) functional health patterns) to help focus nursing intervention on the needs of a young man requiring dialysis. The anecdotal discussion presents the case that Gordon's model has been useful. Murphy uses the discussion to propose the idea that nurses have an important and unique role to play in the care of people requiring dialysis. The paper does present evidence of both the usefulness of Gordon's model and of nursing's uniquely valuable role. By publishing this evidence in the professional press, Murphy is able both to present her case and to ensure that her arguments are made available for critique. It is these last two qualities that ensure the anecdotal discussion does constitute evidence.

The failure to use evidence

Intuition

Intuition is similar to the concept of an educated guess. A simple example of this is where a nurse accepts a new patient on to the ward. The nurse may want to collect a wide range of information from the new patient but this may take time. As a priority, the nurse ensures that he or she finds out just one piece of information – the patient's medical diagnosis. Our nurse takes the view that, with this information, he or she can plan care that is at least broadly appropriate. In this situation, the nurse is using intuition. The nurse takes the medical diagnosis and from this makes inferences about which nursing care is likely to be needed.

Example from the literature and research

Herbert *et al.* (2001) considered the view that evidence-based practice was simply too difficult to apply to the busy clinical arena. They considered the view that clinicians already knew what to do by virtue of their training, established practice, etc. However, after considering the arguments for and against evidence-based practice, they concluded that evidence-based practice did indeed have much to offer the clinical arena.

Too much reliance on intuition can work against the principles of evidence-based practice. Clearly, nursing is not medicine, and our nurse requires information on the patient's nursing needs in order to provide good-quality care. Intuition may be needed from time to time, perhaps in an emergency when there simply is not time to acquire all the information that we would like to have at our disposal. However, the overuse of intuition is an important cause of poor-quality care and it can drive nursing (and medicine) in the opposite direction from health care that is properly based on evidence.

Trial and error

Trial and error is perhaps the worst possible way to improve practice. By definition, this approach lacks methodology or any form of systematic planning. Trial and error involves dealing with a problem by randomly selecting a possible solution. If this solution seems to work, then it is adopted, without seeing whether another solution might work better. If no success is achieved, then the next possible remedy is selected and the process begins again. No attempt is made to see how other practitioners have dealt with the problem. The failure to do this often means that unworkable solutions to the problem are repeated in hospitals and other places around the country and around the world.

Trial and error is perhaps the easiest approach to use because it requires no effort. However, it is dysfunctional, resulting in wasted time and poor patient outcomes. It can never be fully successful. Even if one thinks that a good solution has been found, the possibility will exist that there is an even better solution out there somewhere. It follows that the best possible outcome of trial and error is a good-enough solution. Nursing is an important professional activity, and a good-enough solution can never be justified: it can never be good enough.

Unpublished endeavour

Let's consider a situation where an individual nurse uses research to discover something new or a benchmarking group manages to improve an aspect of practice across several departments. Here, however, the individual nurse researcher or the benchmarking group fails to publish their work. It follows that what has been achieved will not be made subject to review by a wider audience of nurses, and nurses everywhere will not be able to benefit from what has been achieved.

In a sense, the local initiative has managed to base its practice on evidence. However, this is not enough. Nursing is a profession, which means that nurses' responsibility does not start and end with the patient: nurses are responsible for the health and welfare of their profession and have a duty to ensure that knowledge is passed on.

Why is there not more published research in nursing?

It is the case that nursing is a particularly broad (some might say poorly focused) discipline with a history outside mainstream academia. Nursing has a particularly broad focus. It is involved with modalities of traditional care, treatment for those with ill-health and trauma across all age groups and in both institutional and community-based health programmes, the prevention of ill-health and the promotion of health, including psychological, physical and developmental health. In addition, nursing probably still has an image of being an adjunct to medicine rather than an independent professional activity. Funding bodies naturally like to be clear about where they are spending their money. Medicine, with its tight focus on treating disease, presents an easily understood image to the organisations with money to spend on research. Perhaps it is the case that nursing needs to be clearer about what it does and what it aims to do, and to be much clearer about how it presents its image to the general public.

It is worth thinking about this a little more. Imagine the last time you came back from work, tired after a busy day caring for people. Imagine that you were asked what you had done that day, what you had worked on, what you had achieved. If your reply is something like 'Well, loads of things. I don't know *what* exactly, but I know I have been really busy.' Now imagine that the whole of nursing is just like your day has been. Just like you, nursing does not really know what it has done or why; it knows only that it has been busy. Now ask yourself whether this image of nursing is one that would attract research funding. Medicine has a clear focus: we all know what it does – it tries to cure illness and make people better. Nursing does do some amazing things, but perhaps it needs to be clearer about what it does.

Nursing's professional status was, for a time, largely dependent on its association with medicine. In short, and for a variety of reasons, nursing did not freely embrace research but was content to conduct its practice based on custom and tradition (Walsh and Ford 1989a, b, c). In part, at least, nursing remains a little uncomfortable with research, there are no clearly visible funding streams for nursing research, and nursing is perhaps a little less clear than it ought to be about its central focus and purpose. All these factors militate against nursing practice being supported by research and other forms of evidence. However, things are changing and, although there is still much more that can be done in relation to research, nursing does now embrace the principle of evidence-based practice. Nursing is undergoing an evolutionary process in which research will play a central part. In addition, the move of nurse education into the university sector will gradually have the effect of empowering nurses to think about research, to use research and to conduct research themselves.

Perhaps it is the case that the kind of evidence used to support and develop practice is less important than a willingness to use evidence. In the real world of nursing with resources that are often limited, it is sometimes necessary to accept evidence that is second best. This is true of all practice disciplines that deal with human beings. In the long run, however, what matters is a willingness to drive nursing forward, to make things better and to expose new initiatives to one's peers so that those initiatives may be appropriately critiqued and so that others can learn from what we have managed to do. This energy, this wish to take responsibility for the development of our area of practice, is what marks out a profession from other occupational groups. Nurses should never be people who wait to be told what to do; nurses should always be actively developing their own area of work, for patients but also for the whole profession of nursing.

The ethics of research

The history of research in health care is replete with examples of imaginative and heroic endeavour. Medical researchers were often clinicians who indulged in research in their spare time. We owe much of what we know today to early research that was practised on patients' and (often) doctors' own bodies (Trumble and Cavanagh 2006); (Grossman 2008). Although much has been learned from this research, so too has rather too much harm been done. The early researchers of X-ray technology often succumbed to malignant disease secondary to the radiation inflicted on themselves in the hope of discovering more and more about the technology. Sometimes, doctors have been rather too keen to try out their new ideas on patients, who were not always kept fully informed about the dangers inherent in the new technique. Perhaps the worst example of this is that of lobotomy, where 'difficult' patients in mental-health settings had their frontal lobe removed to cause them to become placid and compliant.

Example from the literature and research

Ken Kesey's book *One Flew Over the Cuckoo's Nest* is a novel about the way lobotomy was used to control the behaviour of disruptive patients (Kesey 1962). The novel was made into a film by Milos Forman in 1975.

Example from practice

Charles Grossman (2008) describes the first use of penicillin in the USA. The drug was sent by post from England. When the doctors opened the package, they did not know what to do with the brown substance in the vial, there being no guidance on the matter. The doctors decided to dissolve the contents of the vial in saline and pass the resulting mixture through an asbestos filter in the hope of purifying it. The recipient of the drug was a moribund patient who was suffering from a fulminating infection. The patient survived.

It is sometimes difficult to separate clinical practice, which has as its aim the welfare of one particular patient, and clinical research, which chiefly aims to help future patients. However, there is an important distinction between the two. If you were to go into hospital for treatment, then you would expect that treatment to be wholly directed to your welfare and not be compromised by any expectations that what can be learned from your case might help others. You may well be prepared to be the subject of an experiment, but you would expect to be made perfectly aware that that was what was going on. In practice, it is only too easy for a practitioner to 'just try something out' on a patient, but this is wrong on at least two counts: first, practice should be evidence-based and not 'evidence-generating'; and second, patients have a right to be treated as ill people and not as the subjects of an experiment.

The Royal College of Nursing (RCN) code of research ethics can be downloaded free of charge from the RCN website: **www.rcn.org.uk/**.

Practitioners who carry out research need to regard their two roles as separate. Someone working as a staff nurse has access to patients' records. The nurse does not need permission to read a patient's notes. However, that same nurse, when working on his or her research project, has no right of access to patients' notes; for this, our nurse researcher must obtain consent from the patient and authority from the relevant ethics committee. The two roles of practitioner and researcher are separate, even when practised by the same person on the same day.

The importance of clinical research ethics was highlighted in the mid twentieth century, when doctors (supported by nurses) working for the Nazi regime experimented on civilian prisoners (Lefor 2005). Such experiments included the use of surgery without anaesthesia and exposing people to extreme cold. These events remain today as evidence of the potential of medicine to cause deliberate harm in the name of research and science. In response to this, the Nuremburg Code (1949) and the Declaration of Helsinki (World Medical Association 1964; Williams 2008), adopted in 1964, established the core principles of research ethics. Today, the codes of research ethics published by each professional discipline (Royal College of Nursing 2007) exist to ensure that all planned research is ethically scrutinised.

Principal considerations

- Research is an important way in which nursing and health care improve the quality of its provision.
- All research planning should be subject to oversight by the local research ethics committee and in health care by the system of research governance set up by the government (see the Department of Health website at **www.dh.gov.uk**).

- Research should be well designed and of good quality.

- The research should be justifiable in terms of potential benefits.

- Research should be safe, and any potential to cause harm should be considered in relation to the considered benefits of the research.

- The potential benefits of the research may not necessarily justify exposing participants to risk.

- There should be informed consent.

- Children and vulnerable people present special difficulties, principally in relation to informed consent. It may not always be ethically appropriate for parents and guardians to consent for children.

- Information about participants should be held confidentially and data should be secure.

- Participants have the right to withdraw at any time.

> Your own university will have a research ethics committee. Find out who is the chairperson, go and see them and ask if you can sit in on a committee meeting as an observer. This will be an interesting experience that will teach you a lot about the ways in which research proposals are scrutinised.

Published research will tend to mention research ethics only if ethical considerations have impacted on the design of the research. Often, the published paper will not even mention that ethical approval was given for the study to go ahead. However, one should not be concerned at this. Authors often have very little space in which to communicate their research to the readers and so ethical issues tend to be left out of the discussion. All clinical research and just about every other sort of research as well does have to be approved by the relevant research ethics committee, and it is reasonable to expect that this has been done.

Concluding remarks

In this chapter we have seen that research is not the only mechanism we have for producing new knowledge. In fact, there exists a wide range of other forms of evidence. We have noted, however, that research remains the gold standard and that we need to be careful before accepting other forms of evidence. We have seen that it is not always possible to undertake formal research on people, especially when they are vulnerable and unwell. Thus, we have to ensure that research complies with established ethical principles and guidelines, and so we often have to accept lower forms of evidence. This means that, in practice, the nurse has always to bear in mind that we may not always know things as well as we think we do. It follows from this that the nurse should take available opportunities to improve the quality of existing evidence, whether that means using such tools as audit or benchmarking or of embarking on formal research.

Summary

- It is a principle of evidence-based practice that the practitioner should always be able to defend their practice by identifying the degree to which it is supported by evidence.

- Well-designed research studies provide us with best evidence with which to support and develop practice.

- Good-quality, well-designed research studies are expensive and may be ethically problematic in a discipline that deals with vulnerable people. For this reason, it is often necessary to take recourse to research designs that are less than perfect and to forms of non-research evidence.

- There are several forms of non-research evidence that can be used usefully to support and develop practice. These include such techniques as peer review, exposing ideas to publication and benchmarking.

- Care should be taken in accepting all forms of evidence. Each should be examined logically. Non-research forms of evidence are particularly vulnerable to human error, to bias and to the effect of variables that may be unidentified or poorly understood.

- Of central importance is the nurse's enthusiasm for practice and the desire to make things better. Practice should be founded in evidence, and nurses who are enthusiastic about their work will want to use evidence to support and to develop practice for the good of patients and for the good of the whole profession.

- All research must comply with ethical standards and be approved by the local research ethics committee and in the NHS by the system of research governance set up by the government. Practical guidance on research ethics are published by the various health care professions, including the RCN.

Further reading

This paper looks at the use of peer review (peer observation):

Davys, D. and V. Jones (2007). 'Peer observation: a tool for continuing professional development ... including commentaries by Dominique Lowenthal and Dr. Joanna Jackson'. *International Journal of Therapy and Rehabilitation* **14**(11): 489–493.

This paper discusses the difficulties involved in basing practice upon evidence rather than conventional wisdom. The authors conclude that evidence-based practice is really the only way to go, despite the difficulties:

Herbert, R. D., C. Sherrington, C. Maher and A. M. Moseley (2001). 'Evidence-based practice – imperfect but necessary'. *Physiotherapy Theory and Practice* **17**(3): 201–211.

Here is a paper that looks at the way in which benchmarking can be used to improve practice:

Neill, C. and U. Hughes (2004). 'Improving inter-hospital transfer'. *Paediatric Nursing* **16**(7): 24–27.

This is the reference for the RCN guidance on research ethics:

Royal College of Nursing (2007). *Research Ethics: RCN Guidance for Nurses.* London: Royal College of Nursing.

This paper discusses the ways in which clinical guidelines can be developed through the use of clinical governance:

Stewart, E. (2006). 'Nursing guidelines: development of catheter care guidelines for Guy's and St Thomas''. *British Journal of Nursing (BJN)* **15**(8): 420.

This paper considers peer review:

Yoder-Wise, P. S. (2008). 'The value of peer review: the hard workers behind the scenes'. *Journal of Continuing Education in Nursing* **39**(4): 147–148.

References

Castledine, G. (2008). 'Overzealousness in accident and emergency nursing'. *British Journal of Nursing (BJN)* **17**(18): 1199.

Duncombe, M. A. (1979). *A Brief History of the Association of British Paediatric Nurses 1938-1975*. London: Association of British Paediatric Nurses.

Dyer, I. (1997). 'The significance of statistical significance'. *Intensive and Critical Care Nursing* **13**(5): 259-265.

Gordon, M. (1994). *Nursing Diagnosis, Process and Applications*. St Louis, IL: Mosby.

Grossman, C. M. (2008). 'History of medicine: the first use of penicillin in the United States.' *Annals of Internal Medicine* **149**(2): 135-136.

Herbert, R. D., C. Sherrington, C. Maher and A. M. Moseley (2001). 'Evidence-based practice: imperfect but necessary'. *Physiotherapy Theory and Practice* **17**(3): 201-211.

Jolley, J. (2007). 'Separation and psychological trauma: a paradox examined'. *Paediatric Nursing* **19**(3): 22-25.

Jolley, J. (2008). 'The enlightened sixties'. *Paediatric Nursing* **20**(2): 12.

Jolley, J. and L. Shields (2009). 'The evolution of family-centered care'. *Journal of Pediatric Nursing* **24**(2): 164-170.

Kesey, K. (1962). *One Flew Over the Cuckoo's Nest.* New York: Viking Press.

Lefor, A. T. (2005). 'Scientific misconduct and unethical human experimentation: historic parallels and moral implications'. *Nutrition* **21**(7/8): 878-882.

Murphy, F. (2006). 'Dialysis: a care study exploring a patient's non-compliance to haemodialysis'. *British Journal of Nursing (BJN)* **15**(14): 773-776.

Nuremberg Code (1949). *Trials of War Criminals before the Nuremberg Military Tribunals under Control Council Law*. Washington, DC: US Government Printing Office.

Royal College of Nursing (2007). *Research Ethics: RCN Guidance for Nurses*. London: Royal College of Nursing.

Stewart, E. (2006). 'Nursing guidelines: development of catheter care guidelines for Guy's and St Thomas'. *British Journal of Nursing (BJN)* **15**(8): 420.

Trumble, S. and K. Cavanagh (2006). 'Shades of grey'. *Australian Family Physician* **35**(5): 277.

Walsh, M. and P. Ford (1989a). *Nursing Rituals, Research and Rational Actions*. London, Heinemann.

Walsh, M. and P. Ford (1989b). 'Rituals in nursing: "we always do it this way"... part 1'. *Nursing Times* **85**(41): 26.

Walsh, M. and P. Ford (1989c). 'We always do it this way: rituals in nursing in the surgical area examined in the light of research based evidence'. *Nursing Times and Nursing Mirror* **85**: 26-35.

Williams, J. R. (2008). 'The Declaration of Helsinki and public health ... original declaration reproduced in full with permission of the World Medical Association'. *Bulletin of the World Health Organization* **86**(8): 650-652.

World Medical Association (1964). *Declaration of Helsinki*. Helsinki: World Medical Association.

Xu, W., A. D. Towers, P. Li and J. Collet (2006). 'Traditional Chinese medicine in cancer care: perspectives and experiences of patients and professionals in China'. *European Journal of Cancer Care* **15**(4): 397-403.

Chapter 4
Research methods and design

CHAPTER OBJECTIVES

The objectives for this chapter are to:

- Discuss the need for research studies to be well planned and fit for purpose

- Identify those methodologies that are commonly used and from which originate most other methodological approaches found in nursing research.

Chapter outline

This chapter is about how research is planned and designed.

By now, you will have developed an understanding in your own mind about how research fits with nursing. Let us be clear: this has been quite a journey for you. You have learned a great deal and much now makes sense that did not make sense before. Therefore, you are ready for the next challenge: to make sense of some of the most commonly used kinds of research design.

You have already come across the two most important kinds of research in nursing: quantitative and qualitative research. Now we will look more closely, particularly at quantitative research, in order to identify some of the more important subtypes of research. It is not necessary to know about every kind of research design, but knowing some of the more important ones will be a great beginning and will allow you to make sense of other research methodologies as and when you come across them.

Design and method

Anything good needs to be well planned. Research often requires the invest-ment of a considerable amount of time, and no one wants to waste their time on a badly conceived project. In this, research is just like any other project: it is just like planning to build a new house, for example. Get your house design wrong and you could waste a lot of time and money.

If you do wish to build your own house, you will need to spend some time plan-ning the build. Houses don't just spring up by themselves. More than this, you might want the house to be just right for you and your family, especially if you are spending a lot of time and money on the venture. Building your new house will be quite a project for you and that is exactly what it will be – a project. You will need to design the house. You might want to build a modern house with all the latest labour-saving and energy-efficient gadgets. On the other hand, you might want to build a more traditional-looking house with an emphasis on good-quality materials and that looks fabulous. If you have sufficient funds, you can design the house of your dreams, as long as the design is good. It wouldn't do to build a house that was beautiful but that fell down during the first winter storm. There is more than one possible design but, whatever the design is, it needs to be good and fit for the purpose for which it is intended. In the same way, research needs to be designed, it needs to be planned; there are many available designs, but whichever is used, it needs to be good. Sometimes, researchers sub-stitute the word 'robust' for 'good'. A research design should be robust. That is, it should be fit for purpose, just like your house, and it should withstand any criti-cism, just like your house needs to withstand the winter storms.

You can build your house using one of several available methods. After the Second World War people built lots of prefabricated houses because they needed to build houses quickly (Stevenson 2003). You might wish to have your house hand-crafted from the best wood or you might choose to use bricks or concrete. You will build your house using the method of your choice. In the same way, research studies all employ a method; in other words, the design of the study is implemented, or carried out, using a method.

So, the design of a study is 'what will be done' and the method of a study is 'how it will be done'. When you plan your new house, you will probably plan the design and the method of building at more or less the same time. In fact, that is a good idea. It is just the same with research; indeed, people often use the form 'design and method' together. Sometimes, they like to sound important, so they use the words 'design and methodology'; this sounds much more intellectual. However, we all now know that it means nothing more than the way the research is planned – that is, its design and the methods that are to be used to implement that design. The design and methodology exist as the plan for the research.

Once decided upon, the research will possess a plan (design and methodology), which is at that point a kind of road map of how the research will be executed. It is like the instructions that you will give the builders so that they can build your new house to your exact specifications.

If you are thinking of purchasing an existing house, you will want to know about its structure and how it was built. The same is true of research: the design and methodology of any study are of interest to those who may wish to critique the study. It is important that the design and methodology of the research are available because, unlike a house, which anyone can see, it isn't always possible to tell from data how those data were collected. So, design and methodology are about the planning of research. However, the design and methodology of a study are just as important *after* the study is completed because they allow others to judge the quality of the study.

The elements of research design

There are a range of things that need to be considered when planning any research. These fall conveniently into the following categories:

- *Quantitative or qualitative*: quantitative research tries to identify the facts about something, whereas qualitative research tries to explore and find meaning in something. Usually, quantitative research deals with numbers whereas qualitative research deals with verbal or textual material.

- *Descriptive, experimental and explorative*: descriptive research tries to identify 'what is' or 'what has been'. Experimental research (experiments) is concerned with 'what if' situations to develop new ways of doing things. Explorative research is often qualitative and aims to provide a new insight into things. Sometimes, this is a first step to other forms of research but at other times it is sufficient in itself.

● *The amount of control*: control is arguably more of an issue for quantitative research. The researcher has to make decisions about the degree to which sampling, random allocation and blinding are used.

● *The design*: it may be necessary to have only one group within which data are collected. A survey often has only one body (group) of data. However, an experiment may involve having a control group, for example for reasons of comparison. Designs can be very simple (one group) or they can be quite complex.

New words

Sampling It is not always possible to collect data from everything or every person in which we are interested. In this situation, the researcher will sometimes collect data only from a sample. In this case, steps need to be taken to ensure that the sample is representative of the whole (the population).

Random allocation This is the process by which the researcher ensures that each participant has an equal chance of being selected in the study and allocated to a group (for example, the experimental group or the control group) within the study. It is a way in which an attempt is made to reduce the possibility of bias.

Blinding This is not as brutal as it sounds. Blinding is the process of ensuring that the individuals who provide, collect and interpret the data do not know which group they are in. For example, a patient in a drug trial might not know whether they have been taking the drug or a placebo, and a researcher collecting data from patients might not know whether each patient (participant) has been exposed to the treatment or is in the control group. Blinding is another means of reducing the possibility of bias or the unconscious interpretation of data.

Most of this is just common sense. It can seem complicated because there are a lot of ways in which research can be conducted. We need to have labels for all of these methods in order to communicate them. None of these research methods is difficult to understand; it is just that there are a lot of them. In addition, not all the terms are mutually exclusive; in this way, we can have qualitative descriptive studies but we can also have quantitative descriptive studies. Nevertheless, designing a research study is so common-sense that you could design one now. The section below presents a research problem and asks you to design a suitable study. You will be given prompts so that all you need to do is tick a few boxes. So, let's see whether you can design your own research project.

Design your own study

This study is concerned with the choices made by nursing students at the end of their first year of study. You need to find out how many of them think that they have selected the right field (adult nursing, children's nursing, mental health nursing, learning disability nursing) and how many think that they would like to reconsider their area of specialism. You don't need to explore their feelings on the matter; rather, you simply want to know whether they are happy with their choice or whether they may decide to change to another field.

Now design a study that would be most appropriate. Here are some prompts – just tick the boxes:

Is the study quantitative or qualitative?

Quantitative research tries to identify the facts about something, whereas qualitative research tries to explore and find meaning in something. Usually, quantitative research deals with numbers whereas qualitative research deals with verbal or textual material.

Quantitative   ☐

Qualitative   ☐

Is the study descriptive, experimental or explorative?

Descriptive research tries to identify 'what is' or 'what has been'. Experimental research (experiments) is concerned with 'what if' situations to develop new ways of doing things. Explorative research is often qualitative and aims to provide a new insight into things. Sometimes this is a first step to other forms of research, but at other times it is sufficient in itself.

Descriptive   ☐

Experimental   ☐

Explorative   ☐

Will you take a sample or use all of the end-of-first-year students?

Take a sample ☐

Use all of the students ☐

What design will you use?

It may be necessary only to have one group within which data are collected. A survey often has only one body of data. However, an experiment may involve having a control group, for example for reasons of comparison. Designs can be very simple (one group) or quite complex.

One group ☐

Two or more groups to enable a control ☐

What controls will you design into the research?

Control is arguably more of an issue for quantitative research. The researcher has to make decisions about the degree to which sampling, random allocation and blinding are used.

Will you use randomisation (for selection and allocation to groups)?

Randomisation for selection (if used) of students ☐

Randomisation for the placement of students into experimental and control groups (if used) ☐

No randomisation ☐

Blinding - will you keep any aspect of the research secret from the participants (students) or the people collecting or interpreting the data?

Blinding of participants (so they don't know which group they are in) ☐

Blinding of data collectors or those interpreting the data (so they don't know which group the participants are in) ☐

No blinding ☐

So, how did you design your study? Here are the appropriate answers:

Quantitative or qualitative?

Quantitative ☑

Qualitative ☐

We are collecting data about people's choices. We can do this quantitatively because we do not want to ask the students about their motivation or feelings about which branch to move to.

Descriptive, experimental or explorative?

Descriptive ☑

Experimental ☐

Explorative ☐

This is a descriptive study: it is describing 'what is'. The students have made their decision (or have decided that they are unsure) and we simply need to find out what it is they have decided.

Use a sample or use all of the end-of-first-year students?

Take a sample   ☐

Use all of the students   ☑

We could take a sample here, but we probably want to know what each actual student wants to do.

Which design?

One group   ☑

Two or more groups to enable a control   ☐

We need only one group of students. We don't have a group for each branch. We have one group of students who will tell us which branch they wish to enter. We don't need a control group, because there is nothing to control.

Randomisation?

Randomisation for selection of students   ☐

Randomisation for the placement of students into experimental and control groups   ☐

No randomisation   ☑

There is only one group of students and we have used the whole cohort – so randomisation is not needed.

Blinding?

Blinding of participants (so they don't know which group they are in)   ☐

Blinding of data collectors or those interpreting the data (so they don't know which group the participants are in)   ☐

No blinding   ☑

There is only one group of students. The students can't be blinded because they already know who they are. As there is no control group, blinding cannot be used in relation to the researchers' knowledge of which students are in which group.

The chances are that you either made the same decisions as those listed above *or* you have good reason for making other decisions. Perhaps you chose a qualitative study because you wanted to explore the students' thinking behind their choice of branch. You were not asked to do this, but no one said you had to do what you were told. Indeed, this might make a very interesting study. You may have chosen to use a sample. This might be a good idea if we were interested in generalities, such as what is the likelihood that more students are going to want to change branch this year compared with last year? Sampling may also be necessary if the population of students (that is, all of them) is very large.

So, you have just designed your first research study. You did it with common sense, intelligence and analysis. Whatever we know about research, whatever experience we have, it is most important that we use those very same qualities when designing a study. Knowledge is never enough. The most experienced researcher needs the skills that you have just employed here.

Types of design

One of the reasons why research can seem complicated is the multiplicity of available designs. House building is complicated in the same way: there are just so many designs for houses. Questions inevitably arise as to which design is best, most fit for purpose, most robust, etc. It is not necessary to learn about all the research designs ever conceived. Most professional researchers are familiar with just a few designs that are relevant to their area of research, so it would be unfair to expect you to know more than they do. Rather, it is better for you to learn just one or two designs. Learn these well and they will provide a good foundation for a solid understanding of research. In time you may come across other designs, but these will make more sense, more easily, because you will be able to compare them with the one or two designs you learn now.

Research designs, just like the design of a house, are logical and systematic; they are plain, black-and-white, straight-talking things. You wouldn't want any 'grey' areas in your house design, any places where questions could arise about what exactly you wanted. In the same way, the research design is a deeply practical thing. The design is logically contrived; this means (just about) that it is drawn up using a lot of common sense and a little bit of knowledge.

We have already seen that you could design your own research study, just by using your common sense. However, there are a few kinds of research design of which you need to be aware. Most research in nursing will be planned using one of the designs below:

- *Qualitative*: usually purposed to 'explore' a phenomenon.

- *Quantitative*: there are two main groups of quantitative designs:

  - *Descriptive* (or 'non-experiment'), identifying 'what is' situations. Sometimes descriptive studies have just one group of data, and sometimes there are more than one group so that differences can be identified. However, descriptive studies are retrospective; they measure 'what is' (what has been).
  - *Experimental*, identifying 'what if' situations. These are sometimes called prospective designs because they are producing situations that do not exist at the moment.

We should be clear that there is more than one way to design studies that use one of these main design groupings. However, it is far more important to understand the difference between an experiment and a non-experiment, for example, than it is to understand the several different forms an experiment can take. There is not a 'best' design, although some designs do tend to suit some disciplines and some situations. Medicine tends to use the experimental design whereas sociology tends to use surveys and descriptive studies. Nursing is an eclectic discipline and as such uses a wide range of designs. This does make it really quite difficult to get an overall hold on nursing research. Doctors are much luckier: once they have understood a randomised control trial, they will have learned all they need to know about research. Nurses, on the other hand, have a much harder time of it: there is barely any type of research design that is not used in nursing.

Deductive and inductive research

To deduce something is to reach a conclusion about a question by drawing on one or more general principles. We may, for example, attempt to explain an adolescent's behaviour by using Piagetian theory of human development (Piaget 1952; Piaget and Inhelder 1972). Researchers sometimes do the same thing with their research: they allow existing theory to guide the research (see Fincham and Jaspars 1979). Deductive research is more commonly found in disciplines that have well-developed theories. If you were to ask a psychologist to explain their work, they might say that they were a Freudian psychologist, a cognitive psychologist or a behavioural psychologist. These terms represent major theoretical streams of thought (theories). It is not surprising, then, that a behavioural psychologist might want behaviourist theory to guide each stage of the research process. Researchers are explicit about the theory that has underpinned their research and sometimes write a section of their research report on the theoretical underpinning or the theoretical model that has been used.

Students are sometimes asked to plan a potential research study. Sometimes, these unfortunate students are required to include a chapter on the theoretical model that the student is supposed to use to guide the research. The poor student then thinks madly about what theory they should be using; after all, they have to write a whole chapter on it.

This is all very unfortunate because most nursing students will find that they can't think of any theories and those they do know about simply don't seem to fit their proposal.

This comes about because some people think that nursing should have lots of theories. Psychology and sociology have theories, so nursing should have some too. However, nursing is not psychology; nursing is a practice discipline that deals with facts about practice rather than theories about the universe.

One way for our poor student to deal with this is to write the chapter on 'inductive research' - what it is and how it has shaped the proposal. There: problem solved!

Deductive research is not so commonly found in nursing. Nursing is rightly a pragmatic and practice-focused discipline. It uses a unique mix of knowledge from many different disciplines and arguably does not have theories of its own. If you asked a nurse to explain their work, they might tell you what sort of ward they worked on but it is unlikely that they would explain their work by making reference to a nursing theory. We should not worry about this: it doesn't make us any less clever or any less academic. In fact, medicine is in much the same position: there are no real theories of medicine. Medicine, too, simply uses a unique mix of knowledge from other disciplines such as pharmacology, histology and even nursing. What differentiates medicine from nursing is that the two disciplines use a different mix of knowledge.

Nursing and medicine tend to use inductive research (see Maputle and Nolte 2008). To reason inductively is to draw general principles from detail. In this way, we might look at an adolescent's behaviour and come to a new understanding of adolescence, which we might then use to help us understand the behaviour of other adolescents. Inductive research is a bottom-up approach: it deals with questions about the particular (about practice) and aims to create a new understanding. Indeed, inductive research is often the way in which theory is developed. Nurses and doctors tend to be interested in details about practice. They ask questions such as 'How can we better control procedural pain?' and 'Why do these children appear to be so afraid of injections?' Research into the former may eventually help us to better understand pain itself (we will be developing a new theory of pain). In the second example, research into children's fear of injections may in time help us to understand the way that children construe invasive techniques.

> ## New words
>
> **Variable** Something that varies. A variable can be the thing that is being observed and tested in research. In an experiment, the *independent variable* is the treatment, the thing that is designed to cause an effect on the dependent variable. The *dependent variable* is the thing that reacts to being experimented on. It is the thing in which the effect of the intervention is witnessed and measured.

Qualitative designs

The term 'qualitative' is a little misleading because quantitative methodologies are often employed to look at the quality of something. It is better to consider qualitative methodologies as those that explore feelings, personal interpretations and experiences. It follows that qualitative studies only ever involve people (not planets, motor cars or animals). Also, it is usually the case that qualitative studies collect verbal or written data rather than numbers. This is simply because feelings, personal interpretations and experiences are usually best explored using language rather than numbers. The key here is 'exploration'. We could ask someone to rate their level of happiness on a five-point scale but to explore their perception of happiness using a numerical scale would be difficult. So it is that qualitative studies are associated with some kind of verbal dialogue between the researcher and the participant.

The purpose of qualitative studies tends to be different from that of quantitative studies. In the former, the researcher usually wants to know about one or more people and there is little if any attempt to argue for these people being representative of a population. It is because of this that it is sometimes said that qualitative studies are rather less scientific than quantitative studies. In addition, qualitative studies usually fail the normal criteria for robustness that are applied to quantitative studies. There is no random allocation, no blinding and no means to ensure accurate sampling. However, such concern is misguided, for research is simply a systematic enquiry and qualitative studies are both an enquiry and they are systematic. Qualitative studies are logically determined (well planned) and are focused. Furthermore, qualitative studies address important areas of human existence that could simply not be addressed by quantitative research.

In the past, you will probably have been given a questionnaire like this one:

Module evaluation

How would you rate the module overall?

Poor ☐
Average ☐
Good ☐

Perhaps you look at this and think, 'Well, it was somewhere between average and good.' Perhaps you look at it and say 'But what *is* average? What *is* good? While you can respond to questions like this, you probably value the opportunity to discuss the module with the teaching staff. Such a discussion is more likely to enable you to express just exactly how you feel about the module. The question above is essentially quantitative; the discussion you have with the module leader is essentially qualitative.

Nursing deals with many issues that are better communicated using the rich language that we all possess. In this way, qualitative research often deals with people's experiences that are sensitive, emotive and valuable. It would often be inappropriate to try to put these experiences into prelabelled boxes – and if we did such a thing, we would get a very distorted view of reality.

Qualitative studies are just as focused as any other kind of research. These studies clearly identify the research problem (the focus of the research) and the way in which participants were selected. However, qualitative studies do not usually deal with a sample because there is no population to be sampled. This is because most qualitative studies do not claim that their data are representative of that which might be obtained from other people. In any case, the number of participants (the sample size) tends to be quite small, often fewer than ten people. Such studies are a systematic enquiry into those ten people. Nevertheless, it is important to recruit participants carefully. If the research is focused on patients' experience of pain management, then there would be little point in recruiting patients who had not experienced pain. Because qualitative studies often focus on difficult and traumatic experiences, the search for and recruitment of suitable participants can be a protracted process and one that requires a professionally mature and sensitive approach.

The number of participants recruited in the study is often determined by data saturation. This means that when one begins to obtain the same information from subsequent participants, there is little point in continuing with the data collection. At this point, the data are said to be 'saturated' and the recruitment of new participants is stopped.

There are no experimental and control groups in qualitative studies. Usually, there is just one group of participants, although sometimes two or more groups can be established when a degree of comparison is warranted. Most qualitative studies, however, have only one group of participants.

Most planning decisions for qualitative studies relate to how participants will be questioned. For example, it may be better to interview participants one at a time or to enable a group of participants to discuss questions together (a focus group). It may be necessary to conduct only one interview or several interviews, even many may be needed. As always, the planning for this should be based on what makes most sense in relation to what the research is goaled to explore.

It is the case with almost any research that the researcher hopes to summarise the data and to make the data understandable. In quantitative studies, the researcher might use statistical analysis, which in part works to provide a succinct summary of the data. In just the same way, the qualitative researcher will try to summarise what often amounts to many hours of interview data. In most cases, a form of content analysis is used to create themes or commonalities in the data. These themes may then be presented to the participants as a way of asking them 'Does this summarise what you told me?' Sometimes, the participants will respond, 'Well, no, not really' or 'Well, partly', in which case the researcher will have to do some work on the themes until the participants are happy that they reflect what they said in the interviews. Perhaps you can see that the data collection and the analysis can become merged into one process in qualitative research. This is because the process of providing the data is a learned experience. Participants' understanding of what they have experienced (the focus of the research) can and often does change as they go through the process of communicating that experience. The researcher, too, often becomes part of this process. There is at least a sharing of responsibility for the data between the researcher and the participants, with all parties being committed to producing information that accurately reflects what has been and is being experienced. Much of the planning for qualitative research is focused on these aspects of the study, namely the collection, re-collection and ongoing analysis of the data.

Some common types of qualitative research

Phenomenology

Phenomenology attempts to describe individuals' lived experiences. Phenomenology can look to the outsider as if it deals with the subjective world. However, phenomenologists take the view that what people perceive as real is in fact real and therefore objective to that person. Phenomenology seeks to identify the meanings that people find in their experience, for example of being hospitalised or of giving birth. It is necessary for this meaning to be shared with the researcher, and thus a common understanding is reached.

Example from the literature and research

In a phenomenological study, Rosedale (2009) found that women who had survived breast cancer felt lonely and isolated but that at the same time they developed a deeper relationship with their children and found themselves to be more compassionate and understanding of the suffering of others. The phenomenological orientation of the research study helped to focus the research on the way in which the women found meaning in the way their relationship with others had changed.

Grounded theory research

Grounded theory was developed by Glaser and Strauss (1967) and is inductive in nature, emerging itself in the personal realities of human experience. Grounded theory research is used where no previous research exists. In this way, grounded theory research is used to explore new areas of human experience. Grounded theory does not use existing theoretical frameworks but aims to generate a new theory of the aspect of human experience being examined.

Ethnographical research

Ethnographical research developed from anthropology. Ethno means 'people' (as in 'ethnic') and graphic means 'drawing' or 'picture'. Ethnographic research focuses on culture (a particular culture or an aspect of culture) and examines peoples' behaviour within that culture or the differences between two cultures. Just like anthropologists, ethnographical researchers will immerse themselves in the culture being examined and will seek to become accepted by the people they wish to study. The researcher will then identify participants who are willing to talk about the aspects of their lives that are central to the culture in question. Ethnographic research concerns itself with such diverse cultures as those of remote tribes or that of nursing in the UK.

Qualitative research can be particularly interesting and does have the advantage (for some) that it rarely involves any statistical analysis. The output of qualitative research can be easier to understand than that of quantitative research. In many ways, qualitative research seems to suit nursing, which after all has a focus on care and on human experience.

Example from the literature and research

Using an ethnographical approach, Roberts (2008) worked within the culture of nursing to examine the ways in which student nurses helped each other to learn. The research found that students formed friendships with other students and that these friendship groups were used to provide peer support for learning

Quantitative designs

In some ways, quantitative designs seem harder to understand than qualitative designs because there are so many of them. For this reason, we need not worry about identifying every type of design. To do that would be very tedious and would not be much use. Instead, let's look at the main forms that quantitative designs take. Your enthusiasm for nursing, together with your intelligence and your common sense, will enable you to adapt these as necessary. In addition, you will gradually learn about new designs as you read more about research and as you begin to practise research.

The survey

A survey has a single group of participants, such as a sample of people eligible to vote at the next election. A survey is also descriptive: it aims to describe one or more aspects of the sample. For example, a survey may aim to describe how people claim they intend to vote at the next election. A survey is not an experiment because there is no independent variable. Our survey would become an experiment only if, for example, we showed one group of participants a film (the independent variable) of how poor university students had become, before asking them how they might vote at the next election. We might then compare the results from this group with those from a control group who had not been shown the film about impoverished university students.

A survey may be simple, but sometimes it is exactly the right choice. At some point, you will have been asked to evaluate a module or course of study at your university. In this case, the university simply wants to know what its students think of the course; it wants to use standard questions with closed, multiple-choice-like responses. For this, a survey is both simple and perfect.

Module evaluation

How would you rate the module overall?

Poor	☐
Average	☐
Good	☐

New words

Differences and correlations Often we want to consider the difference between one set of data and another set of data, and most statistical procedures are designed to do this. Sometimes, however, we want to determine the degree to which one set of data agrees with or matches another. For example, as children grow older, they tend to grow taller; indeed, age and height in childhood do correlate positively.

The survey design is so simple that you might wonder why one should ever use anything more complicated. However, on the whole, we can only analyse survey data descriptively. This means that we can calculate descriptive statistics such as counts and percentages but we cannot easily determine differences or correlations between two groups of data. So, a survey is good for describing what is, usually from one group of data. If this is what we want to do and we are sure we won't want to do anything else, then a survey is perfect.

Although a survey usually has only one group of data, it is sometimes possible to split the data into two or more groups. For example, a survey of potential voting behaviour could look for the existence of differences between male and female voters. This may be reasonable where we are simply attempting to describe 'what is' in relation to the sample as whole. However, we may quickly run into problems with the sample size for males and females if we do not select the sample with a view to studying the variable sex. Also, we would really need to ensure that the sampling procedure we used was capable of selecting an unbiased sample of both men and (separately) women. In practice, it would be a good idea to have deliberately set out to study the voting patterns of men and women, rather than to decide to do so after we have generated the data.

Planning is important. Of course you could design and build your house with three bedrooms and then decide to add another bedroom later. However, people will always know that that room was added later; you will never get the colour and style of brick to match that used in the rest of the house. It is just like that with research. It is rarely possible to get away with bad planning. If we want to look at the voting behaviour of men and women and how men and women vote differently (if they do), then we should design our research for this purpose - and if we did, we would probably choose not to use a survey.

The descriptive design

The word 'descriptive' is used here largely for want of a better word. However, what we mean here is a design that is not a survey because it has more than one group designed into it but it is not an experiment because it seeks only to describe 'what is'. A descriptive design does not have an independent variable because it is not seeking to test out something new. Some people call this sort of design 'retrospective'; this is another label meant to indicate that such studies aim to look at 'what is' (or, really, 'what has just been') situations. Descriptive research does not manipulate situations to study them; experiments do.

Descriptive studies lack some of the controls that can be put in place for experiments (prospective designs). In this way, there is no randomised control study for the descriptive design. It is not usually possible to have such controls in a situation where the researcher is studying what is already taking place. Perhaps, for example, we wish to look at two different nursing procedures in respect of how much pain they may cause. In this situation, the nursing procedures have been practised for some time. It isn't possible to set up a control because all of the patients in this situation simply have to have one procedure or the other. However, some controls can be put in place. We may be able to provide a degree of randomisation in relation to the selection of participants and the allocation of them to groups. We could ensure that the person collecting the data is not aware of which procedure the patient had (blinding). Perhaps we could even ensure that the patient didn't know which procedure he or she had. In practice, however, these controls can be very difficult to apply to descriptive studies. It is a little like us having built our house, only then to decide that it would be good to put in an environmental monitoring facility to measure how energy-efficient the house is. We could probably do this, but it would certainly have been easier to have planned this into the design of the house from the beginning. The descriptive design is used where 'the house' is already built. That is the situation with which we are dealing; we can't undo the fact that 'the house' is already built.

There may be a tendency to criticise descriptive designs for the lack of control they are able to apply. However, randomisation, blinding and control groups may all be quite impossible to apply here. In practice, few if any research studies that involve human participants can ever be perfect. It is perhaps important only to make each study as robust as possible. The material that descriptive studies concern themselves with is the 'what is' situations of life as they are being played out today. It is often important that we research what happens today in nursing. Such studies sometimes lead in time to further experimental studies that can offer better control and that can develop new practices for the future.

The experimental design

We are all familiar with the notion of an experiment. It conjures up images of white-coated scientists messing about with test tubes over a Bunsen burner. This is actually a rather useful image because it is in the laboratory that experiments are most easily undertaken.

New words

Control group A group exposed to no treatment at all in order to determine what effect the treatment has.

Experiment Formally, an experiment is said to exist where the researcher introduces one or more independent variables to determine their effect on one or more dependent variables. However, the experimental design is also associated with studies that require a high level of control and with measures designed to ensure objectivity and freedom from bias.

Retrospective Relating to a descriptive design. The opposite is prospective, a term used for experiments.

In the laboratory, it is possible to have control over everything that happens. We can put mixture *a* into test tube *b* and do whatever we want with it. So, a high degree of control is one of the factors that characterise an experiment. It is not usually possible to acquire the same level of control when doing research with people.

The other main characteristic is that an experiment is dealing with novel situations. The researcher will be asking 'what if' questions such as 'What will happen if I mix substance *a* with substance *b*?' So, an experiment is associated with a high degree of control and it deals with new situations. An experiment is trying to discover things about future possibilities; in other words, it is prospective.

It is one thing to run an experiment in a laboratory but quite another to experiment with people. Nursing tends to be interested in people more than it is interested in the content of test tubes. In this, the discipline of nursing is akin to the social science disciplines of psychology and sociology. Human beings are difficult to control. We can imagine all kinds of interesting experiments with people, but the people concerned may not be prepared to be experimented on or may have views about their role within the experiment. Another major issue with experiments on people is that people are inherently variable. They change from day to day and from moment to moment. The laboratory scientist can control all or most of the variables so that they vary only when he or she wants them to; this is rarely possible when working with people. For this reason, experiments with people are rarely perfect.

New words

Randomised control trial A form of experimental design characterised by a high degree of control of the variables and of the data. As the name suggests, a randomised control trial (often abbreviated RCT) will employ random allocation and at least one experimental and one control group.

Experimental or independent variable In experiments (quantitative studies), the experimental or independent variable is the thing that is thought to affect another variable. So, for example, if we measure the effect of giving or not giving a drug for pain, the giving or not giving the drug would be the experimental or independent variable. The resulting pain level would be the dependent variable.

Medicine often uses experimental designs. However, medicine's experiments most often involve drug trials. Here, variables are relatively easy to control. It is probably fair to say that outside drug trials, medicine has the same problem with experiments as does nursing.

Examples of research designs

Let us look at the variety of designs available in quantitative studies. We will start with the simplest designs and gradually begin to look at some more complex ones. The more complex designs often offer better control and are therefore more robust. However, bear in mind that sometimes a more simple design may be perfectly appropriate. If there were a best design, then everyone would use it and we would have to learn only that one design. When planning research, it is important to use the most appropriate design, and that often means using a simple one.

In Figure 4.1, there is just one group. Let's assume that this is a group of people who have been exposed to a nursing procedure associated with pain.

Figure 4.1 Research design for a single group

There may be a lot that we want to find out about these people and their pain. However, let's assume that for the moment we simply want to find out how much pain these people are experiencing after they have been exposed to the nursing procedure in question.

So, this is our design. The x stands for treatment, which is research language for the intervention to which the research participants are exposed. In this case, it is the nursing procedure that we think may be associated with pain.

The Post-test box signifies the collection of data. Perhaps the research will involve the administration of a questionnaire that asks the participants to rate their pain on a scale of 1-10. The term 'post-test' is used to indicate that this comes after ('post') the intervention (nursing procedure) and that it is a 'test', meaning a collection of data.

This design is similar to that of a survey. First of all, it is descriptive; this is not an experiment. The reason that it is not an experiment is that we are measuring only what is already there. We are not introducing a new variable. Second, we have only one group of participants. However, we have selected participants who have had or are having the nursing procedure in question. Surveys often use selection procedures, which can be quite focused and sophisticated. After all, there is no point in asking babies how they will vote at the next election.

Let's remind ourselves of what this study aimed to achieve – a measure of the amount of pain experienced by people who were exposed to the nursing procedure. This simple design should be sufficient. However, there are some things that this design would *not* enable the researcher to do. Think about it now and list below some limitations of this design. You don't need to know the answer to this question; you can use reason and analysis to work it out.

....

....

....

This design will not enable us to work out:

- whether these participants had pain before the procedure;
- whether their pain before the procedure was the same as the pain after the procedure;
- whether the pain was made better or made worse by the procedure.

However, this is not a problem, because the design was intended only to enable the study to determine the amount of perceived pain experienced by the participants after they had been exposed to the nursing procedure. Simple designs can be used to achieve simple outcomes. Indeed, it would be wasteful of resources to enable a design that would tell us more than we needed to know.

More complex designs

Let's look at that list above again:

- Whether these participants had pain before the procedure
- Whether their pain before the procedure was the same as the pain after the procedure
- Whether the pain was made better or made worse by the procedure.

It is often the case that we want to find out whether an intervention makes a difference. Clearly, we could do this by adding a pre-test group. If we test the sample for pain before and after the intervention, then we will be able to determine what effect the intervention has had on the participants' pain (Figure 4.2).

Pre-testing	x	Post-testing

Figure 4.2 Research design using a pre- and post-test group

Remember, X is the intervention, the effect of which we are examining. Exposure to X (the nursing intervention) is the independent variable. The participants' perceived pain is the dependant variable. So, this should do it. Now we are testing the participants' pain both before and after the intervention (a nursing procedure). This should enable us to determine the effect on perceived pain of the intervention. This is sometimes called a 'pre-test-post-test' design. This design may be perfectly adequate. It will tell us:

- whether these participants had pain before the procedure;

- whether their pain before the procedure was the same as the pain after the procedure;

- whether the pain was made better or made worse by the procedure.

But research needs to be robust and resistant to criticism. Take another look at our pre-test–post-test design and see whether you can see a potential flaw in it.

We know that pain can be remedied by a wide range of things. We know that anxiety can increase pain and that reassurance can reduce pain (Oshodi 2007). Perhaps it is possible that the pre-testing might have the effect of reassuring the participants that they are cared about. After all, they haven't even had the procedure yet and someone is already asking them whether they have any pain. The mere presence of someone spending time with the participant and asking about their welfare might just enable them to cope with the procedure better.

Example from practice

McDougall *et al.* (2006) used a pre-test–post-test design to evaluate a community paediatric outreach team's effectiveness in relation to the care of children with acquired brain injury.

So, perhaps our design would be better if we had another group of participants who did not have (were not exposed to) the pre-testing. Then we could be sure that the pre-testing was not influencing the results from the post-testing.

So here we go. In Figure 4.3, we have a group of participants who do not have the pre-testing.

| (a) Pre-testing | x 1 | (b) Post-testing –1 |

| x 1 | (c) Post-testing –2 |

Figure 4.3 Research design using three groups of participants

We probably now expect to see a difference between (a) and (b), but there should be no difference between (b) and (c). If there is a difference between (b) and (c), then we would suspect that the pre-testing has had an undesirable effect on our data. We should note, however, that this design is more expensive, because this design will need a third more participants and the researchers will have to do one more testing. We should also bear in mind that we may simply not have available sufficient participants to enable the use of this design.

However, we are not through yet because we can think of another problem with our design. You may be wondering where the control group is. You are right: there could indeed be a problem with our design.

But why would we need a control group? After all, we can tell what happens between pre-testing and post-testing; surely whatever difference exists must be due to the intervention. Perhaps so, and there may be times when a control group is not warranted. A control group is going to be expensive and we shouldn't use one if we can make a convincing argument that it isn't needed.

Anyway, let's look at what a design with a control group can look like. The design in Figure 4.4, sometimes known as the Solomon four-group design (see Chapman and Richman 1998), can tell us:

(a) what difference exists before and after the intervention (experimental group 1);

(b) whether pre-testing is influencing post-testing scores (experimental group 2);

(c) whether the difference found in (a) would have occurred even without the intervention (control group 1);

(d) whether the effect found at post-testing was simply due to the passage of time (control group 2).

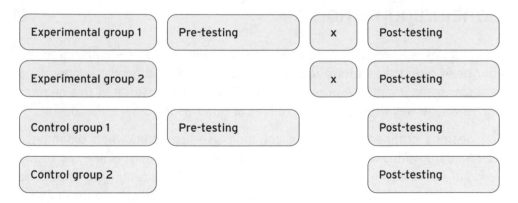

Figure 4.4 Research design using control groups

If our researchers think that they do not need to test for an effect caused simply by the passage of time or of the effect of pre-testing, then a more simple design may be appropriate. Figure 4.5 shows a design sometimes referred to as the 'classic experimental design'.

Figure 4.5 Classic experimental design

There is no hard and fast rule about whether one needs to test for a particular effect, such as that of time (the passage of time) or of pre-testing. With each research project, it is necessary to make informed choices about what should be tested. Sometimes a more simple design is perfectly appropriate, and at other times a more complex and costly design is necessary. Perhaps the Solomon four-group design, with its ability to test for just about everything, is as close to perfection as we can usually get. However, it may test for things that are surplus to requirements and in so doing may make an unwarranted use of other people's time and money. Both time and money are often precious resources. A great deal of health research is funded by charitable income, and researchers have a duty to use the available funding wisely. For this reason, there is no perfect design, just a most appropriate one in a given situation.

Concluding remarks

This chapter will probably have presented you with some new material to get your head round. If you have found this chapter a little difficult to understand in places, read it again. A good understanding of the material in this chapter will serve you well when you come to look at other aspects of research.

The designs outlined here are in common use. However, when planning a research study, it is always necessary to create a design that is specific to the needs of the research study in question. There is no best design; nor should we choose a design just because it happens to be popular. When you design your house, you will not choose the most popular design, for you will want your house to be just as you want it to be. Your house may have to be energy-efficient or it may have to withstand storms or floods. Perhaps your house will need to keep out the heat of the day and be capable of collecting every last drop of rain. There is no best design, only a design that is fit for purpose and that does the job intended of it. So it is always necessary to think and use one's intelligence and imagination, just as you have been doing as you have read this chapter.

Summary

- Research needs to be well planned. The planning is called the 'design and methods' of a study.

- The plans need to be available after a study is complete, so that others can see how the study was undertaken and judge its quality.

- There are many designs used by research in nursing, and these can look complex, largely because there are so many of them. This simply reflects that nursing is a broad discipline. The many research designs in use reflect the fact that nurses have become interested in a wide variety of phenomena and the many different ways in which patients' lives can be improved.

- There is no perfect design, only a design that is most fit for purpose in relation to the aims of any one particular research study.

- In determining the most appropriate design, the researcher needs to think carefully about what is to be achieved, what constraints exist and the degree to which any proposed design will produce a robust study.

Further reading

Examples of quantitative studies:

Meyers, T. A., D. J. Eichhorn, C. E. Guzzetta, A. P. Clark, J. D. Klein and E. Taliaferro (2004). 'Family presence during invasive procedures and resuscitation: the experience of family members, nurses, and physicians ... reprinted with permission from the *American Journal of Nursing*, 2000;100(2):32-42'. *Topics in Emergency Medicine* **26**(1): 61-73.

Terry, L. M. and J. Carroll (2008). 'Dealing with death: first encounters for first-year nursing students'. *British Journal of Nursing (BJN)* **17**(12): 760-765.

Example of a phenomenological study:

Rosedale, M. (2009). 'Survivor loneliness of women following breast cancer'. *Oncology Nursing Forum* **36**(2): 175-183.

Example of grounded theory research:

Drury, V., K. Francis and Y. Chapman (2008). 'Mature learners becoming registered nurses: a grounded theory model'. *Australian Journal of Advanced Nursing* **26**(2): 39-45.

Example of ethnographical research:

Roberts, D. (2008). 'Learning in clinical practice: the importance of peers'. *Nursing Standard* **23**(12): 35-41.

Example of a descriptive study (this one is qualitative):

Mackintosh, C. (2007). 'Making patients better: a qualitative descriptive study of registered nurses' reasons for working in surgical areas'. *Journal of Clinical Nursing* **16**(6): 1134-1140.

Example of a deductive study

Fincham, F. and J. Jaspars (1979). 'Attribution of responsibility to the self and other in children and adults'. *Journal of Personality and Social Psychology* **37**(9): 1589-1602.

Example of an inductive study:

Maputle, M. S. and A. Nolte (2008). 'Mothers' experiences of labour in a tertiary care hospital'. *Health SA Gesondheid* **13**(1): 55-62.

Example of experimental research:

Edwards, H., A. Walsh, M. Courtney, S. Monaghan, J. Wilson and J. Young (2007). 'Improving paediatric nurses' knowledge and attitudes in childhood fever management'. *Journal of Advanced Nursing* **57**(3): 257-269.

Example of explorative research (this one is qualitative):

Jeong, S. Y. and D. Keatinge (2004). 'Innovative leadership and management in a nursing home'. *Journal of Nursing Management* **12**(6): 445-451.

Examples of randomised control studies:

Jubb, R. W., E. S. Tukmachi, P. W. Jones, E. Dempsey, L. Waterhouse and S. Brailsford (2008). 'A blinded randomised trial of acupunture (manual and electroacupuncture) compared with a non-penetrating sham for the symptoms of osteoarthritis of the knee'. *Acupuncture in Medicine* **26**(2): 69-78.

Harkin, C. and R. Parker (2007). 'A prospective, randomised control trial of acupuncture for select common conditions within the emergency department'. *Journal of Chinese Medicine* (85): 41-48.

Example of a survey:

McCabe, A. and H. Duncan (2008). 'National survey of observation and monitoring practices of children in hospital'. *Paediatric Nursing* **20**(6): 24-27.

References

Chapman, M. V. and J. M. Richman (1998). 'Practice highlights: promoting research and evaluation of practice in school-based programs: lessons learned'. *Social Work in Education* **20**(3): 203-208.

Fincham, F. and J. Jaspars (1979). 'Attribution of responsibility to the self and other in children and adults'. *Journal of Personality and Social Psychology* **37**(9): 1589-1602.

Glaser, B. G. and A. Strauss (1967). *The Discovery of Grounded Theory: Strategies for Qualitative Research*. Chicago: Aldine.

Maputle, M. S. and A. Nolte (2008). 'Mothers' experiences of labour in a tertiary care hospital'. *Health SA Gesondheid* **13**(1): 55–62.

McDougall, J., M. Servais, J. Sommerfreund, E. Rosen, J. Gillett, J. Gray, S. Somers, P. Frid, D. Dewit, L. Pearlman and F. Hicock (2006). 'An evaluation of the paediatric acquired brain injury community outreach programme (PABI-COP)'. *Brain Injury* **20**(11): 1189–1205.

Oshodi, T. O. (2007). 'The impact of preoperative education on postoperative pain: part 1'. *British Journal of Nursing (BJN)* **16**(12): 706–710.

Piaget, J. (1952). *The Origins of Intelligence*. New York: Harcourt Brace.

Piaget, J. and B. Inhelder (1972). *The Psychology of the Child*. New York: Basic Books.

Roberts, D. (2008). 'Learning in clinical practice: the importance of peers'. *Nursing Standard* **23**(12): 35–41.

Rosedale, M. (2009). 'Survivor loneliness of women following breast cancer'. *Oncology Nursing Forum* **36**(2): 175–183.

Stevenson, G. (2003). *Palaces for the People: Prefabs in Post-War Britain*. London: Batsford.

Chapter 5
The nature and collection of data

Chapter outline

In this chapter we will look at data, what they are and how they are collected. 'Data' is a collective term for the stuff that is collected by research. In this chapter we will look at what form data exist as before they are made subject to statistical or qualitative analysis. The fact is, not all data are the same. Of course, there are data that exist as numbers and data that exist as written or spoken words. However, a quick look at the different forms of data will bear much fruit later on in terms of our understanding of analysis and in relation to our understanding of research in general.

Once we have spent a page or two looking at the different kinds of data, we will be able to relax a little and briefly consider the various ways in which data can be collected.

What are data?

Numerical data

Essentially, data are the stuff that is collected during a research project. The data will be made subject to analysis. Data can exist in the form of numbers (in quantitative research) or as words (in qualitative research).

> ### New words
>
> **Raw data** Data before they are analysed - the actual stuff collected by researchers.
>
> **Datum** A single piece of data, like a single number. The word 'datum' isn't found much in the literature, but the plural from 'data' gives rise to some rather odd sounding sentences such as 'the data were analysed'.

So why are data important? Why not just look at results? We can just look at the results of a study, but understanding the kind of data used will help us to make sense of the results. There are different kinds of data, and the kind of data used in a research study will determine the kind of analysis that is used. Let's look at some of the things that you know:

Qualitative data usually exist in the form of words, sometimes written words, sometimes spoken words, but words in some form or another. We cannot easily use statistics with words. We cannot ask, for example, what is the average of 'happy' and 'sad', and we cannot easily add happy to sad. So, some forms of analysis fit with some forms of data and not with other forms of data.

There are some forms of analysis that do not work with some forms of numerical data. So, we can add up the number of males and we can add up the number of females. Let us say that there are 15 men and 15 women in our sample - so then the average sex is '15'? You already know that that doesn't make sense. So, there are some statistical procedures that cannot be used with some forms of data.

The sort of data we have fit with the analysis that is required. Understanding this can help us to make sense of the analysis. When a research project is planned, the researcher will identify the kind of data that the study will produce and will then identify the appropriate analysis. This is important because not every kind of data can be analysed as we might want - remember, however big our sample, even if we were able to sample every male and every female in the world, we will never be able to calculate an average sex because there will always be just so many males and so many females.

This is more serious than it sounds; look at the next example: Let us say that we want to measure the amount of pain experienced by patients after they have sustained a fractured femur. Foolishly, we ask 1000 patients: 'Do you have any pain?' We find that 999 patients say 'Yes' and one says 'No' (that patient had actually come into hospital for an eye test but had accidentally joined the queue of patients with a fractured femur because he couldn't read the signs well enough).

So, how much pain did the patients have? Well, we don't know; we asked them only whether they had pain. These kind of 'yes/no' data do not give us very much information, even though we have a sample of 1000 people. In circumstances like this, people say that the data are not 'rich' or not 'deep'.

It is worth bearing in mind that if we collect 'shallow' data, we may not be able to do much with them. You may think that no one would be daft enough to choose to collect such shallow data, but you would be wrong to make such an assumption. When you read the research literature, you should question whether the data collected really were the best that could have been collected. Nurses collect data all the time as they assess patients and clients and make decisions about them. Imagine that you can see one of the 999 patients being admitted to an orthopaedic ward. Look at the nurse who kindly and sympathetically approaches his or her new patient and asks 'Have you any pain?' Oops!

So how should we ask patients about their pain? Well, of course you know how to do that. In fact, you will probably have used a pain scale of some sort or another. Figure 5.1 shows a pain scale that is often used with children.

Figure 5.1 Wong-Baker FACES Pain Rating Scale

Source: Hockenberry MJ, Wilson D, Winkelstein ML: Wong's Essentials of Pediatric Nursing, ed. 7, St. Louis, 2005, p. 1259. Used with permission. Copyright, Mosby.

So now we have a scale; in this case, the scale is quite short (0–5) but it still allows us to:

- determine a mean score for pain;[1]

- develop at least some idea of whether there is a little pain or a lot of pain;

- determine differences between groups of people in relation to pain; for example, we can determine whether pain worsens or improves with a nursing procedure.

Some scales are longer than one to five. These longer scales can give us richer information. Imagine, for example, that your sphygmomanometer[2] gives readings only between 1 and 5. You will agree that that would not be a good thing. Sometimes a patient's systolic blood pressure (BP) may be as low as 40 mmHg (this patient is clearly not very well) or as high as 250 mmHg (this patient is not very well either). That's quite a big scale. In fact, the scale on which we measure BP doesn't really have any ends to it; it can even be negative – like the pressure in the veins in your legs if you were to hang yourself upside down like a bat. Perhaps we could simplify the scale, but would you want to do that? It can be quite useful to know that the patient's BP has gone up from 40 mmHg to 45 mmHg – at least the patient is improving. Apparently minor moves up and down a scale can be important. So, sometimes long scales are useful as they offer seriously rich data.

We have seen that some forms of data give us more information than do other forms of data. Not all data are the same. We have used numerical examples here, but exactly the same is true of qualitative data. Here, we can ask someone whether they have pain, and we record the verbal response, 'yes' or 'no'; or perhaps the patient will say 'I have a little niggle' or 'My big toe really hurts when I walk on it'. These responses are qualitative data. Try adding up three little niggles

---

[1] The mean should be used with care when the scale is not continuous. The mean in this case could be returned as 5.5 (for example) or a number half way between 5 and 6. Yet, it is not possible for a patient to choose such a number.

[2] A sphygmomanometer is a blood-pressure recording machine.

and a big toe - it just doesn't work - but the responses are data all the same, they have meaning to us, meaning that is shared between the patient and ourselves. These data exist as a common understanding. However, the data are pretty shallow and most qualitative researchers would turn up their nose at such a form of enquiry (Baker 2006). The qualitative researcher is more likely to ask 'Tell me about your pain' or perhaps 'How do you feel when you have pain?' (Whiting 2008). Such questions are likely to yield data that are rich (or deep).

Types of quantitative data

Researchers are fairly objective people (some would say that they can be fairly concrete too). We have been talking about shallow and rich data, but researchers like to nail these concepts down. We have three main types of numerical data:

- *Categories* - called 'nominal' data
- *Small scales* - called 'ordinal' data
- *Long scales* - called 'interval' or 'ratio' data.

These four terms, nominal, ordinal, interval and ratio, are sometimes referred to as 'levels of measurement' (Vojir *et al.* 2006). They are really levels of data. Interval and ratio are deeper levels (rich in information), and nominal is a relatively shallow level, offering less depth of data. Here are some examples:

Nominal level of measurement – categories

- Yes/no questions
- Discrete categories, such as are you male or female? Are you tall, middle-sized or short?

Sometimes, a range of categories can look like a small scale:

Normally, do you drink:

(a) No alcohol

(b) Up to two units of alcohol per day

(c) More than two units of alcohol per day?

In practice, however, a scale with fewer than five points on it is usually regarded as categorical (as discrete categories and not as a scale). It would be possible to calculate a mean from the data produced by the alcohol question above, but the result would not be quite as meaningful as we might like. If we assigned numbers 1, 2 and 3 to the responses, we might find that our 'average' score was (for example) 1.5 – that is, somewhere between 'no alcohol' and 'up to two units per day'. However, we would need to bear in mind that no one would have given such an answer. In this way, the average score did not really reflect the raw data.

Nominal level data have a range of statistical procedures available to them, which tend not to be used on ordinal, interval or ratio data. An example of such a statistical procedure is the Pearson chi square, which can be used to test for differences between, for example, two groups of categorical data, in the form:

Particular preference for wearing a uniform	Yes	No
Females	12	4
Males	5	12

In this completely fictitious example, 17 males and 16 females were asked whether they wanted to wear a uniform or to wear their own clothes at work. We can see here that there is a relationship between the responses given by males and females. Males in this fictitious example were more likely to respond 'no' and females were more likely to respond 'yes'. The data here are categorical – that is, they exist in categories and are therefore at the nominal level of measurement. Perhaps the data here are not very rich or deep; we don't, for example, know why our fictitious males wanted to wear their own clothes at work or the strength of feeling they had on the matter. However, these data are useful here. Sometimes categorical data are all that we have available to use – males are males and females are females and that is that. Sometimes, categories do tell us all we need to know about something. Statistical procedures such as the Pearson chi square are available for use on categorical data. In fact, if we ran a Pearson chi square on the data here, we would get the result 5.155, with $p = 0.0232$.[3] Don't worry about the numbers just yet; they mean, however, that the difference we see here between the responses of males and females is not likely to be due simply to chance – that is, it is not a chance finding. Some people would describe this result as 'significant'.

[3] Chi square with Yates correction, two-tailed.

So, Pearson chi square can work for nominal level (categorical) data. Not all statistical procedures work here though. Consider one of the most simple statistical procedures, the mean or average. Try to apply the average to the data in the preference for wearing a uniform box above; you will probably not make much useful progress.

Ordinal level of measurement – ranking and short scales

The ordinal level of measurement is so named because it is meant to be used with a list of possible responses that are placed in order - that is, they are ranked. Here is a list of things that the research participant could be asked to order:

What causes you most pain? Please place in order, with [1] at the top of the list causing most pain.

- Getting up in the morning

- Walking

- Running

- Having to bend down

- Having to move after a period of sitting or resting

Such ordinal lists can give us some quite useful information (data). In practice, however, the lists are usually quite short. Imagine having to place in order a list with 100 items on it. On the other hand, these ordinal lists are longer than those we looked at in the nominal level of measurement. In a way, these lists form a short scale. This is important because, over the years, a range of statistical procedures have been developed for ordinal lists that work just as well for any short scale.

Short scales are often used in research, largely because research participants find them easier to work with than they do with longer scales. Perhaps the most commonly used short scale is a Likert scale.[4] A Likert scale presents the research participant with a statement and then asks the participant to choose a response from a list. Here is an example:

I think that NHS dentists should be available to everyone:

1. Strongly disagree

2. Disagree

---

[4] First proposed by Rensis Likert (1903–1981).

3. Neither agree nor disagree

4. Agree

5. Strongly agree

The data resulting from this short scale are probably best analysed using a range of statistical procedures designed for the ordinal level of measurement. This is the case, even though such short scales do not require ranking (placing in order).

Ordinal level data have a range of statistical procedures that have been designed just for them. An example is the Mann–Whitney U statistical procedure, which is used when we want to test differences between two groups of data, each produced using a short scale (ordinal level data) (Crichton 2000).

Interval level of measurement – long scales

Your essays are probably marked on a scale from zero to a hundred. This is quite a long scale. In fact it is so long that it is effectively continuous. It is true that you (probably) cannot be awarded a score of 55.789%, but there are so many points in the scale 0–100 that points between any two numbers would be meaningless to most of us.

These longer scales provide richer data. If your academic work was marked on a scale of one to five, you might begin to be dissatisfied with the meaningfulness of the mark. You might, for example, want your university to distinguish between those people who got a 'lower three' and those who 'nearly got a four'. There is no correct length of scale for every purpose. We have to determine for ourselves what length of scale produces data that are meaningful to us and what length gives us the richness of data that we think is appropriate.

Degree classifications are usually of the form:

- First class

- Upper second class

- Lower second class

- Third class

- Pass

This seems to work well for most people. However, the poor student who gets one mark under a first-class degree (usually 70% overall) might well feel unhappy that the overall percentage mark is not printed on their degree certificate.

There is no perfect length for a scale. It is up to us to determine what length of scale is fit for purpose. However, it is always the case that longer scales give us more information. Interval level data have a rather larger range of statistical procedures available to them than is the case for either nominal (categories) or ordinal (short-scale) data. This reflects the increased richness of interval level data. We would probably not use the Mann–Whitney U procedure for two groups of data as we did for ordinal (short-scale) data; rather, we might use a procedure called the Student's t test. Don't worry about all these statistical procedures just yet, but do bear in mind that different kinds of data often require different statistical procedures. It is not important to be able to remember which statistical procedure fits with which kind of data, but it is useful to understand that not all data are the same and that at some point we will need to be sure that the most appropriate statistical test is used.

Ratio level of measurements – long scales without any ends

Relax: this chapter has got as difficult as it is going to get. We have already come across ratio data. These are simply data that have no top and no bottom. We have noted that blood pressure can be below zero sometimes and can be as high as you like. You can't get more than 100% for your examinations because those data are interval and have a known bottom (0%) and a known top (100%). However, data in the form of blood pressure, body temperature, bacterial counts and blood alcohol have no limits. In practice, a bacterial count of –1 is a little difficult to construe, but at the top end it can be just about anything. Blood pressure over 500 mmHg is probably not compatible with life. However, there is a real difference between these scales and the one used for your examinations. Ratio level data do exist. But we noted that things were not going to get any more complicated, and they won't. Effectively, and in practice, interval and ratio level data are treated exactly the same. If we know interval level data, then we know ratio data, and the statistical procedures used for one can be used with the other.

Numbers – summary

Just a little effort with the question of the different types of numerical data (numbers) will help a lot with our grasp of research in general. Numbers can be confusing. However, let us review what we have learned here.

There are essentially four levels of data:

- *Nominal*: categories, such as yes/no
- *Ordinal*: ranked data or short scales, such as a Likert scale
- *Interval*: longer scales, where the middle ground between say 57% and 58% is effectively meaningless
- *Ratio*: just like interval data but without a known top and bottom to the scale.

These levels are important because they relate to:

- the richness of the data;
- the choice of statistical tools available to us.

Researchers are sometimes limited to a particular level of measurement (such as ordinal) where the data only ever exist at that level. However, sometimes researchers can select data-collection tools that will yield data at a particular level of measurement. In this way, the researcher can require the participant to respond with 'yes' or 'no' or can use questioning with a short or a long scale. In this case, the choice is important because it relates directly to the range of statistical procedures available to the analysis and the 'amount' of information that the data are able to yield.

Types of qualitative data

Qualitative data take the form of words or meanings. The data can be taken from written communications or verbal dialogue but can also take the form of still or moving images, ideas, drawings and anything that is capable of being summarised and interpreted. Some people will question the scientific nature of qualitative data, but it is suggested here that qualitative data can be and are handled scientifically. In addition, we have noted already that qualitative data are often used to explore situations that could not be explored quantitatively.

However, numbers can be used to explore meanings. In fact, we have already come across an example of this:

I think that NHS dentists should be available to everyone:

1. Strongly disagree
2. Disagree

3. Neither agree nor disagree

4. Agree

5. Strongly agree

This is a Likert scale. It is being used here to obtain data on people's views on the provision of NHS dentistry. In this example, a number is being assigned to a notion, idea or viewpoint. This can work well when we know what the notions, ideas or viewpoints are. It probably works well here. We know what range of views exist about the provision of NHS dentists, or we can at least take an educated guess at what views exist. In essence, the research participants, the data collector and the data analyst are all likely to be speaking the same language; they understand each other. So, a whole range of feelings, emotions, experiences and all things human can be and often are explored quantitatively – using numbers.

Qualitative research comes into its own when, basically, we don't know what questions to ask and where a shared and meaningful communication with the research participant is not at all straightforward. Nurses are often interested in the things that make their patients and clients psychologically uncomfortable. These things often exist as experiences that trouble the patient or client in some way. Consider, for example, the experience of having a child in the intensive care unit (ICU), or the experience of someone who is in grief or distress.

If we could know how parents felt about having a child in the ICU, then we might be better able to help them. The trouble is, most of us don't know what it is like. We can guess, but most of us would be conscious that we might guess incorrectly. We are often quick to suggest that we don't know how someone else feels. It can be difficult to 'get inside someone's head' and see things the way they see them. Qualitative research is good at exploring feelings, notions, experiences, etc., which we don't know very much about.

Not only do we not know what the individual is feeling but also we know so little about it that we don't even know what questions to ask. Structured questions seem particularly inappropriate. Consider the following questions asked by our fictitious nurse admitting a child to ICU. The questions are directed to the child's mother:

- How old is Benjamin?

- Is he on any special diet?

- Does he have any special words (e.g. for 'toilet') of which we should be aware?

And then:

- Are you not anxious ☐, a little anxious ☐ or very anxious ☐?

- Do you think that Benjamin will die? Yes ☐, No ☐

Of course, this is not appropriate: the nurse would not ask these questions and neither would the researcher. There are two reasons for this:

- We do not know what the child's mother is experiencing, so we don't know what to ask her about.

- Even if we think we know what sort of things she is experiencing, we are uncomfortable about putting these into preconceived or artificial categories. In this example, we do not know whether Benjamin's mother is thinking about his possible death; she may not have construed events in this way. There may be other thoughts that are important to Benjamin's mother and that it would be useful to know about. In asking Benjamin's mother about death, the nurse is putting thoughts inside the mother's head. Here, the nurse is impacting on the mother's construction of reality. In clinical practice, this is not good; in research, it is very damaging. We want to know what the mother is thinking about, not what she is thinking about after ideas have been suggested to her by a third party.

In asking these questions, we run the risk of insulting the participant or patient, in the way that our question can suggest an answer. One does not ask 'Do you think that Benjamin will die?' without suggesting to the mother that this is something she *ought* to be thinking of. Clearly, the researcher and the nurse should want to find out what is going on in the participant's head, not what the researcher can put there.

In practice, the nurse would be sensitive about his or her own lack of knowledge of what is going on in the mother's mind. Being so sensitive, she might ask:

- Tell me how you feel.

- Is there anything that you would like to say to me just now?

Questions such as these might enable the child's mother to communicate her feelings freely and without being constrained by artificially contrived questions. The nurse and the child's mother can potentially come to a shared understanding of what is being experienced. This is exactly the way it is with research.

So, qualitative research does have a useful purpose (Wiart and Burwash 2007). It is widely employed in nursing, perhaps because nurses often want to reach a better understanding of their patients' and clients' experiences. It follows that the data in qualitative research are usually focused on human experience. These data usually take the form of words, either spoken or written, but they can take any form from which interpretations can be discerned. For example, when Benjamin begins to get better (which he really did), the nurse might give him paper and pencils and Benjamin might explore his own feelings through drawings (Matsumori 2005; Jolley 2010). Benjamin might find this easier than speaking because he still has an endotracheal tube in his airway or perhaps because, being only four years old, he's not so good at expressing the nuances of his experience in words. Once again, the researcher may well use the same approach – children's drawings have been used to help explore their experiences of violence, of war and of serious illness (Hatlevig 2006; Jolley 2010).

Ways of collecting data

When one begins to look at published research, it soon becomes apparent that data are collected using a variety of means. However, understanding this is easy because you are already aware of these different means.

Here are some of the most popular ways of collecting data. Note that, in each case, the method of collecting the data influences the kind of data that are obtained:

- Questionnaire

- Interview

- Participant and non-participant observation

- Existing data and meta-analyses

- Historical data and records

- Audio, film and photographic records.

It is important to understand that although there are advantages and disadvantages associated with each type of data collection, there is no right or wrong way to collect data. As with every other aspect of research, there is no right or wrong way to do this, only the most appropriate way, considering what it is that the research project in question aims to achieve. It is worth emphasising this point because people new to research are sometimes too ready to criticise a research project on the basis that the use of interviews, for example, carries some disadvantages. Interviews *do* have disadvantages, but they may still be the best and perhaps the only way of collecting data in respect of what a particular research project is trying to achieve.

Let's look at each data collection method in a little more detail.

The questionnaire

You will probably be familiar with questionnaires. Most of us occasionally receive them in the post or online, get stopped in the street to answer questions or have come across questionnaires at some other point. Almost by definition, a questionnaire is a written thing containing one or more kinds of question. The questionnaire may be presented on paper or increasingly may be available electronically. The questionnaire is simply a means of communication, often used because data can be collected efficiently and inexpensively. It is not difficult to post out thousands of questionnaires to people, who will then (we assume) sit patiently, complete the form and obediently post it back to us. In the same way, Web-based questionnaires can easily reach many thousands of people. In this case, the data can be collected electronically and even analysed automatically. So, let's be clear about this: questionnaires can be very useful. Indeed, it is for this reason that they are so much in use.

Questionnaires can contain questions designed to yield nominal (categories), ordinal (short-scale) or interval (long-scale) data (Rattray and Jones 2007). Here are three questions that deal with each in turn:

> (Q1) Are you male ☐ or female ☐ ?
>
> (Q2) Place in order of preference the following activities:
>
> Watching the TV ☐
>
> Walking ☐
>
> Playing your favourite sport ☐
>
> Going to the gym ☐
>
> Sunbathing ☐
>
> (Q3) What is your yearly income (state amount) [£_____] ?

So, questionnaires are pretty good at delivering data at all the levels of measurement discussed earlier in this chapter. However, questionnaires can also be used to obtain qualitative data, as in:

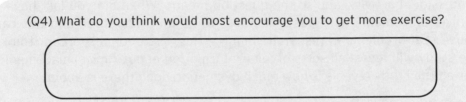

(Q4) What do you think would most encourage you to get more exercise?

Now, some people would regard this as merely an open-ended question. The term 'qualitative research' is probably best left to situations where meanings can be shared between at least two people. The question here is open-ended: the participant can answer as he or she pleases but the question does still have structure (the question could have said 'Tell me what you think about exercise') and, importantly, there can be no dialogue between the researcher and the participant. In qualitative research, it is important to achieve a shared understanding of what is being communicated. A questionnaire can never fully facilitate this because it is not possible for the researcher to probe the partici-pant. Let us say that a participant has responded to question 4 as follows:

(Q4) What do you think would most encourage you to get more exercise?

I hated sports and physical education at school and that has put me off doing any form of exercise now.

Now, it might be good to explore this with the participant, but a questionnaire does not make such an exploration easy. Arguably, questionnaires are best used to collect data from closed or structured questions or when achieving a common understanding with the participant is relatively unproblematic.

You may have had experience of a questionnaire that is hard to understand. If you have had to apply for a UK passport recently, you may be familiar with the problem. It is important that the questions in a questionnaire are meaningful, both to the participant and to the researcher. Consider this question, included in a fictitious questionnaire to student nurses:

(Q5) When did you last experience a period of praxis?

Well, what do you think: is this a question about the menstrual period? Dysmenorrhoea, perhaps. Not really: 'praxis' means the practical side of professional activity, and so the question means 'When did you last have a clinical placement?' It is easy for words to be misunderstood and this can cause real problems in research. Imagine this: the poor researcher thinks the study will reveal all sorts of juicy information about clinical placements, but all the study reveals is how much dysmenorrhoea there is about.

The main disadvantage of questionnaires is that there is often no facility to interact with the participant. However, questionnaires can be used during face-to-face meetings. Sometimes these exist simply to ensure that all sections of the questionnaire are completed and that the participant understands the questions being asked. When someone stops you in the street and asks you for a few minutes of your time to fill in a questionnaire, the chances are that the researcher will complete the questionnaire. There may be only a limited dialogue between the researcher and the participant, but it is sufficient to ensure that the participant understands the questions.

There is another problem that is sometimes associated with the use of questionnaires: we cannot always tell whether the participants have been truthful. There are all manner of reasons for why people don't always want to tell the truth. An individual might not be too truthful about how much exercise they get each day, how much alcohol they drink or when they first had sex. After all, these questions can be perceived as personal. In practice, participants can leave questions unanswered if they don't want to answer them, but all too often they may give us a response that is not true. Researchers don't usually talk about 'truth'; rather, they use the word 'validity'. There are ways in which one can test the validity of questionnaire data. One might ask the same question twice but re-worded slightly, or one might repeat a question on another occasion. A lot is written about validity. The fact remains, though: it is difficult to discern whether a participant lies reliably (consistently). This may be a problem with any kind of data collection, but it is perhaps more of a problem where the researcher and the participant are not working together, as in the case of a postal questionnaire.

On the whole, questionnaires are useful and there are many occasions when they work well. However, as with any kind of data collection, one always needs to question whether there might be a better way of collecting the data. Whether there is or not will usually depend on what the research project in question is trying to achieve.

The interview

This one-to-one communication gets round a lot of the problems associated with the questionnaire. A one-to-one dialogue can ensure that what is communicated is understood by both parties – that is, that there is a common understanding. The interview also enables a less structured, more flexible and more in-depth gathering of data. The interview makes it possible to probe the participant (but not physically!). In the best interviews, the participant and the researcher share a common goal of reaching a common understanding of the participant's views or experiences.

The main disadvantage of interviews is that they are time-consuming and resource-intensive. However, the interview should not be dismissed just because it is resource-intensive. If the interview is the most effective way of collecting data, then interviews should be used. The real question is whether the data could be collected more easily or less expensively in some other way. As always, whether it can or not will depend on what the research study is aiming to achieve.

The interview is probably best used where a shared understanding has to be worked at and where a shared understanding does not come naturally or easily (DiCicco-Bloom and Crabtree 2006). It is not surprising, then, that the interview is often used in qualitative studies. Having said that, interviews are often appropriate in quantitative studies too. Consider the admission interview or pre-admission interview often undertaken by nurses. Here, the nurse asks the patient questions about a range of things, from current health status to who will look after the dog when the patient comes into hospital. Now, it would be possible to send the patient a pre-admission questionnaire, but there are advantages in seeing the patient, not least because it allows any concerns to be probed.

Let's emphasise this point one more time - there is no perfect method of collecting data, only the most effective method in relation to what the study in question aims to achieve.

Participant and non-participant observation

So far, we have looked at methods of data collection that rely on participants' accounts of something that has taken place or on their views or experiences of something. Sometimes, however, the researcher will want to make a direct observation of something that is taking place. So, for example, it is possible to watch health-care staff washing their hands between procedures in order to take an objective measurement of the standard of hand-washing.

'Participant observation' is a term used to describe a situation where the researcher is involved in the situation being measured; in this case, the researcher would be a nurse who would be washing his or her hands, along with the other staff. The nurse researcher might do this 'covertly' (secretly), although these days covert data collection raises a number of ethical concerns and does not tend to be practised. Usually, then, the staff being watched know that they are being watched and have agreed to this. Non-participant observation takes place when the researcher is not involved directly in the practice being measured.

Both participant and non-participant observation can raise concerns about something called the Hawthorne effect[5] (or sometimes performance bias). The Hawthorne effect is where the behaviour of those being watched changes because they know they are being watched. In the case of our nurses, for example, we may find that they take extra care to wash their hands according to the hospital procedure. There are a number of ways to counter the Hawthorne effect, the most usual being for the researcher to be present for some time before data are actually collected. In this way, the behaviour of the individuals concerned eventually returns to normal as they become used to (habituated to) the presence of the researcher(s). Cutler and Davis (2005) used this technique when measuring the quality of oral hygiene performed in intensive care.

The Hawthorne effect is an example (in a sense) of participants being less than honest with the researcher. We have come across this problem before when we looked at the use of questionnaires, but we have perhaps seen here that the problem of honesty pervades most kinds of data collection. In a sense, we do not entirely escape the problem, even where we may, for example, want to count bacteria on nurses' hands as a measure of their hand-washing skills. The bacteria are not going to club together in one heap just because they know they are being watched, but we do have to consider how reliable has been our sampling of the bacteria. So, validity (the extent to which the data are the data we think they are) and reliability (the degree to which the results would be the same if we did the research again) are related concepts at the heart of any research study. Every research study needs to address the degree to which the study can demonstrate validity and reliability. There are ways of measuring validity and reliability (Salmond 2008), but these are far from perfect and each research study should be critiqued in relation to what risks exist that the data may not be what we think they are.

Participant and non-participant observation are resource-intensive means of collecting data. Typically, the process will involve months of work with the participants even before the data collection begins (see Cutler and Davis 2005). There are ethical considerations in watching people and recording what they do, and today's media-sensitive NHS does not always welcome researchers who wish to carry out these modes of data collection.

Participant and non-participant observation remain useful techniques in nursing research and where we want to study the behaviour or performance of nurses or patients. Again, let's make the point that it is not a case of which data collection type is 'best' but rather which mode of data collection is most appropriate, considering what the research project in question aims to achieve.

[5] The Hawthorne effect is so named because it was first identified in studies that took place at the Hawthorne Works, a factory outside Chicago. The effect was first described by Henry Landsberger.

Existing data and meta-analyses

It has always been possible to take existing data and subject those data to analysis. Sometimes the data from existing studies are re-analysed, either to check on the original analysis or to run a different analysis. More usually, data that have not already been analysed will be used. An example of this is the analysis of census data, which take place in various studies (Doran *et al.* 2003). Another example is the use of existing hospital records (Ansell *et al.* 2007). In both of these examples, the researchers in question have not had to collect their data as such. This means that there are fewer ethical issues with which the researchers have had to deal, though there may still be concerns over the researchers having access to the data, confidentiality and whether the data are likely to be held securely and eventually published.

Using existing data is not only a convenient route to data collection; it is also the most appropriate route in situations where the data already exist. It would be a waste of time collecting new data when existing data are available.

An important and relatively new way of using existing data is in the meta-analysis associated with systematic reviews. Systematic reviews have been mentioned in Chapter 4 and are a review of existing research on a particular topic, together with an analysis of the pooled data from (often) several studies. We noted in Chapter 4 that a convenient source of systematic reviews is the Cochrane Library.

Example from the literature and research

An example of a systematic review is that by Stevens *et al.* (2004). This study examined the evidence that the administration of sucrose to neonates could act as a safe analgesia. The systematic review examined the range of existing studies that met set criteria for methodological quality, pooled the data from these studies and subjected the new data set to analysis.

Historical data

Any profession such as medicine or nursing has history. In part, it is the historical depth of the discipline that gives it its professional feel. Understanding the history of nursing makes it possible for us to put the present in perspective. Our understanding of history also helps to prevent us from making the same old mistakes over again and makes it possible for us to learn from what has gone before (Jolley 2006). Apart from all of this, the history of nursing can be a fascinating area to study.

Historical studies can involve searching through archives (Hilton 2005), or they can involve speaking with older people to find out what kind of things happened in the past.

> ### Example from the literature and research
>
> Jolley (2007) interviewed older people who either worked as children's nurses or who were child patients between 1920 and 1970 in order to examine their different perspectives of hospital care in that period.

Concluding remarks

The somewhat dry nature of data is perhaps one reason why people sometimes find that research is not for them. But let's be honest: this chapter wasn't difficult to understand. You may have come across one or two new words, but other than that it was all pretty easy. There is a learning curve at work here. However, if we can understand the different forms that data can take, then we will find that such knowledge illuminates our study of the other aspects of research. If you have been unsure of this chapter, read it again. What has been discussed here is not difficult to understand, but it is important that you understand it.

So we now know that there are different forms of data (levels of measurement). Numerical data exist as nominal (categories), ordinal (ranking or small scales), interval (long scales) and ratio (long scales without ends). As we move from nominal through to ratio, the data become deeper or richer - that is, they contain more information. Researchers need to acquire data that are at least rich enough to be fit for purpose. We have also noted that different levels of measurement (nominal, ordinal, etc.) fit with different statistical procedures. All this needs to be taken into account when research is planned.

We have looked briefly at qualitative data and seen how they can be used to help us measure such things as experiences, feelings and points of view. Qualitative data are much used in nursing and so are appropriate, considering nursing's historical focus on the human aspects of care.

From time to time, we have used examples of the way in which nurses ask questions. We can use such examples to define research because there really isn't any difference between nursing practice and nursing research. In clinical practice, the nurse is always asking questions and working to solve problems. So it is with research: nursing practice and nursing research are simply two sides of one approach to care. One side without the other would be untenable. Just as nursing is focused on care, so too is nursing research. The data collected by nursing research are designed to inform us about the things that most concern nurses – things such as pain, anxiety and discomfort. Data may not seem to be much fun, but when they are used within research they come alive. Data are amazing because of the way they tell us about nursing and because of the way they can answer our questions – and by doing this, data can help us to make things better.

Summary

- Qualitative data usually exist in the form of words rather than numbers. They are often derived from the researcher's attempts to explore feelings and emotions.

- Not all quantitative data are the same. The levels of measurement – that is, nominal (categories), ordinal (short-scale) and interval/ratio (longer-scale) – are important to understand because they determine both the depth of the data (potentially, how much the data tell us) and what statistical procedures can be used on the data.

- There isn't a best sort of data. Sometimes qualitative data better suit the purpose of the research than do quantitative data. Whatever form the data take, the data should fit the overall aim of the research study.

- The kind of data generated by a study must be linked both to the planned analysis and to the specific objectives of the research. It follows that thought must be given to the sort of data that the study will generate at a time when the design and methods of the study are being decided.

Further reading

An introduction to qualitative research:

Smythe, L. and L. S. Giddings (2007). 'From experience to definition: addressing the question "what is qualitative research?"'. *Nursing Praxis in New Zealand* **23**(1): 37-57.

The argument for the full legitimacy of qualitative research:

Wiart, L. and S. Burwash (2007). 'Qualitative research is evidence, too'. *Australian Journal of Physiotherapy* **53**(4): 215-216.

A guide to critiquing quantitative research:

Coughlan, M., P. Cronin and F. Ryan (2007). 'Step-by-step guide to critiquing research: part 1 - quantitative research'. *British Journal of Nursing (BJN)* **16**(11): 658-663.

A guide to critiquing qualitative research:

Ryan, F., M. Coughlan and P. Cronin (2007). 'Step-by-step guide to critiquing research: part 2 - qualitative research'. *British Journal of Nursing (BJN)* **16**(12): 738-744.

An interesting account of a nurse's early experience of being involved in qualitative research:

Katsuno, T. (2006). 'Being a qualitative researcher in nursing'. *Japan Journal of Nursing Science* **3**(1): 5-7.

A research paper showing the use of the chi square and the Mann-Whitney statistical procedures to test the effectiveness of acupuncture:

Jubb, R. W., E. S. Tukmachi, P. W. Jones, E. Dempsey, L. Waterhouse and S. Brailsford (2008). 'A blinded randomised trial of acupunture (manual and electroacupuncture) compared with a non-penetrating sham for the symptoms of osteoarthritis of the knee'. *Acupuncture in Medicine* **26**(2): 69-78.

An introductory paper about questionnaire design:

Meadows, K. A. (2003). 'So you want to do research? 5: questionnaire design'. *British Journal of Community Nursing* **8**(12): 562-570.

A more advanced paper about questionnaire design:

Rattray, J. and M. C. Jones (2007). 'Essential elements of questionnaire design and development'. *Journal of Clinical Nursing* **16**(2): 234–243.

A paper about research interviews:

DiCicco-Bloom, B. and B. F. Crabtree (2006). 'The qualitative research interview'. *Medical Education* **40**(4): 314–321.

An example of a systematic review and the use of existing data in new research:

Stevens, B., J. Yamada and A. Ohlsson (2004). 'Sucrose for analgesia in newborn infants undergoing painful procedures'. *Cochrane Database of Systematic Reviews 2004* (3): CD001069.

A paper on historical research methodologies:

Sweeney, J. F. (2005). 'Historical research: examining documentary sources'. *Nurse Researcher* **12**(3): 61–73.

References

Ansell, P., D. Howell, A. Garry, S. Kite, J. Munro, E. Roman and M. Howard (2007). 'What determines referral of UK patients with haematological malignancies to palliative care services? An exploratory study using hospital records'. *Palliative Medicine* **21**(6): 487–492.

Baker, L. (2006). 'Ten common pitfalls to avoid when conducting qualitative research'. *British Journal of Midwifery* **14**(9): 530–531.

Crichton, N. (2000). 'Information point: Mann–Whitney test'. *Journal of Clinical Nursing* **9**(4): 583–583.

Cutler, C. J. and N. Davis (2005). 'Improving oral care in patients receiving mechanical ventilation'. *American Journal of Critical Care* **14**(5): 389–394.

DiCicco-Bloom, B. and B. F. Crabtree (2006). 'The qualitative research interview'. *Medical Education* **40**(4): 314–321.

Doran, T., F. Drever and M. Whitehead (2003). 'Health of young and elderly informal carers: analysis of UK census data'. *British Medical Journal* **327**(7428): 1388.

Hatlevig, J. (2006). 'Children's life transition following sexual abuse'. *Journal of Forensic Nursing* **2**(4): 165-174.

Hilton, C. (2005). 'The clinical psychiatry of late life in Britain from 1950 to 1970: an overview'. *International Journal of Geriatric Psychiatry* **20**(5): 423-428.

Jolley, J. (2006). 'The progress of care'. *Paediatric Nursing* **18**(8): 12.

Jolley, J. (2007). Separation and psychological trauma: a paradox examined'. *Paediatric Nursing* **19**(3): 22-25.

Jolley, R. (2010). *Children and Pictures: Drawing and Understanding.* Chichester: John Wiley & Sons.

Matsumori, N. (2005). 'Ask the expert: use of the drawing technique in nursing assessment'. *Journal for Specialists in Pediatric Nursing* **10**(4): 191-195.

Rattray, J. and M. C. Jones (2007). 'Essential elements of questionnaire design and development'. *Journal of Clinical Nursing* **16**(2): 234-243.

Salmond, S. S. (2008). 'Taking the mystery out of research: evaluating the reliability and validity of measurement instruments'. *Orthopaedic Nursing* **27**(1): 28-30.

Stevens, B., J. Yamada and A. Ohlsson (2004). 'Sucrose for analgesia in newborn infants undergoing painful procedures'. *Cochrane Database of Systematic Reviews 2004* (3): CD001069.

Vojir, C. P., K. R. Jones, R. Fink and E. Hutt (2006). 'Scientific inquiry'. *Journal for Specialists in Pediatric Nursing* **11**(4): 257-259.

Whaley, L. and D. L. Wong (1987). *Nursing care of Infants and Children.* St Louise: Mosby.

Whiting, L. S. (2008). 'Semi-structured interviews: guidance for novice researchers'. *Nursing Standard* **22**(23): 35-40.

Wiart, L. and S. Burwash (2007). 'Qualitative research is evidence, too'. *Australian Journal of Physiotherapy* **53**(4): 215-216.

Chapter 6
Analysis

CHAPTER OBJECTIVES

The objectives for this chapter are to:

- Demonstrate that little or no knowledge of mathematics is required
- Provide the reader the opportunity to practise doing some data analysis
- Demonstrate that processing numbers with a computer is no more difficult than using words with a word processor
- Introduce the ways in which qualitative data can be analysed
- Illustrate the ways in which qualitative analysis is objective and rational.

Chapter outline

This chapter will look at the use of analytical tools to describe data and to demonstrate the effect that one variable may have on another. The notion of probability will be introduced using examples with which you will probably be familiar. In fact, you will find that you are already fully conversant with the notion and use of probability. Using practical examples, this chapter will demonstrate the use of probability within research. The notion of proof will be examined, and it will be suggested that research seldom proves anything but merely determines the degree to which the results can be trusted.

One of the most scary aspects of research is the statistical analysis that is so often equated with research. This chapter will show that, in fact, very few mathematical skills need to be acquired in order to perform statistical tests.

This chapter will also look at the way in which qualitative data are analysed and will emphasise the very practical, simple and logical decisions that are made about how best to achieve an analysis of non-number data.

What is analysis?

Let's think about your essays for a moment. Perhaps you have been asked to avoid making your essays too 'descriptive'. You may have been encouraged to make your writing 'a little more analytical' or to 'use more analysis'. So, what is analysis? Taken literally, the term 'analysis' means to break something down into its component parts for the purpose of understanding them better. In practice, analysis is the sense that we make of things. It is often the case that when we examine something, we have to pare away the irrelevant material so that we can see the relevant stuff more clearly.

Let's use the example of individualised care and the difficulties that exist in implementing it. Let's say that we want to examine the degree to which individualised care is something that is seen as positive and useful by patients and clients of the NHS. Let's look at some of the component arguments:

- Patients appreciate a nursing service that adapts to their own needs.

- Patients are irritated by a nursing service that seems to be more about the needs of the institution than their own needs.

- The public expects higher standards of nursing care than in the past. As part of this, people expect their individual wishes and needs to be accommodated by the nursing staff.

- Nursing is the provision of care to an individual. Such a one-to-one orientation is fully professional and is something that nursing should be encouraging as part of its effort to be seen as a fully professional service.

These arguments are pretty convincing. However, do these arguments present the whole story? Can you think of some reasons against the use of individualised care? List them here:

1. _____

2. _____

3. _____

4. _____

Here is what you may have written:

All this stuff on individualised care is well and good, *but* it is just not realistic because:

- nurses are too busy;

- nurses don't have the time to modify every procedure for each individual;

- patients should be grateful for what is being offered – the NHS is a charity after all;[1]

- if people want individualised care, they should obtain private treatment;

- nurses don't work for individual patients: in practice, they work for a ward or unit. Nurses work as a team. Their orientation to the ward and the team means that they work together with other people and so can't make individual exceptions to their care with every patient.

So here we have two sets of arguments in mutual opposition. We can't leave it like this, because nursing has to do something, it has to operate in one direction or another, it has to practise individualised care or generalised care.

We are not short of evidence, we have all the evidence here. What we are short of are analysis and synthesis. In analysis, we separate out the various arguments or components. In synthesis, we create a new position. By collating the various arguments and by categorising them (in this case, into 'for' and 'against' groups) we have achieved an analysis; in short, we have broken down the issue into its component parts for the purpose of understanding them (analysis).

Synthesis? What synthesis? No one has ever asked me to put synthesis into an essay.

The word 'synthesis' is often subsumed by the word 'analysis'. In this way, when people use the word 'analysis', they often mean analysis and synthesis.

[1] Actually, the NHS is not a charity, although it may manage charitable organisations and funds.

Doing this analysis has made things clearer. We have two groups of people - nurses and patients - who have a quite separate orientation to the provision of health care. Indeed, patients and nurses are not working together; even their aspirations for what the NHS can provide is in conflict. However, let's firm up our analysis to make it clearer, more succinct and more focused:

- Patients are interested only in themselves; they want care that is focused on their needs. Patients appreciate that other patients also have needs, but their own core role is to obtain the health-care provision that they need in order to get well. That is why they are in hospital or are receiving care. When well, these same patients may fill their life with helping others. Now, though, it is time for them to receive care. It is a question of focus and priority. The purpose of being in hospital is to receive the care that they (themselves) need.

- Nurses are loyal to their ward or unit and to the team of people with whom they work. They are conscious of patients' individual needs but are chiefly orientated to the generalised care that is provided (to all patients) on their ward or unit. This is good-quality care and is made better through it being a team activity. This provides a system in which all patients receive a fair percentage of the time the nurses have to offer and in a situation where resources are often short. To be clear, nurses work for their ward; they do not work for any one patient.

So, this is an analysis of the situation. It is an analysis with which you are free to disagree. An analysis is not necessarily the truth. You may have a different analysis, but in forming this you would have to assemble some more evidence or identify where the analysis here has been illogically construed.

So, perhaps this is interesting, perhaps it even sheds new light on your understanding of individualised and generalised care. Perhaps you have been practising nursing for one, two or three years but only now feel that you understand this issue. Well, if so, you will understand the use and the power of analysis.

So, what about synthesis? Perhaps you have written an essay that presents all the available arguments but does not come to a conclusion, except perhaps to say 'Here are all the available arguments'. Consider a student who has reviewed the available research on a particular topic and found that some of the research evidence is conflicting. Our student summarises the available research but fails to come to a conclusion because the research itself is contradictory. The world is full of contradictory evidence, but when it comes to the practice of health care we have to synthesise all of this conflicting evidence so that it makes sense, so that as practitioners we know what to do. Synthesis is to take separate elements and to create a new whole from those elements. Theory, as in 'a theory of child development', is constructed largely from synthesis. Let's have a go at synthesis with our individualised care issue:

We cannot deny that nurses practising generalised care have done a good job over the years. Such a system is efficient and makes good use of resources. In addition, nurses like it; they like working for an institution (the ward or unit) rather than for individual patients, and they like being part of a team. However, times change and the public's expectation for health care has changed. Not only do patients want individualised care; it is also good for them because they get from the system just what they need. When, for example, they are fit to be discharged home, they go home and do not have to wait until their take-home drugs come up to the ward with all the other drugs, tomorrow lunchtime or teatime or maybe not at all. There are those who would like to see nursing achieve a more professional orientation to their work. From this source has come care-planning, the nursing process and academic nursing itself. We have to decide whether nursing is still institutionalised, whether it exists to serve the hospital or NHS trust, or whether it exists to serve the patient.

Tick only one box in the table below. When you were younger and anticipating your nursing career, did you see yourself primarily:

Working for a hospital or NHS trust	
Working for an ill person	

So, in synthesising this issue, we find that we have to make a decision. We have to decide whether our core priority is to the sick person or to the NHS. We understand now that we cannot be wholly orientated to both the NHS and the patient. Furthermore, we understand that for nursing to progress professionally, it must adopt the patient, for a professional nursing relationship can only ever be between one practitioner and one ill person. With this synthesis we have a new nursing ideology, one that is wholly orientated to the care of just one individual, where responsibility cannot be diffused among the whole ward staff and where the nurse must always be clear what health-care provision he or she is dealing with. The old-fashioned nurse, working for the ward, where patients either toe the line or get in the way, is (in our synthesis of this issue) a dinosaur in a passing age.

But what about all those numbers and complex statistical tests?

Relax! I could ask you how your word processor produces words on the screen and checks your spelling and grammar or how it is that anyone could possibly learn to write in such a complex language as English. Part of this you simply don't need to know and part of it you will learn; there's no hurry. It has been said before in this book that you are amazing. If you can write an essay using such complex language and technical skills, then you can do anything. Certainly, there is nothing in research that you will find difficult.

Try not to be put off by the amount of material on analysis and statistics; no one knows it all anyway. All you have to do is learn the little piece of that knowledge that you need today. As the days add up, you will learn more and more, and that will happen all on its own and without much trouble. It is the same with nursing practice. You might wonder what you learned on your latest clinical allocation, but by the end of your course you will know heaps of things. Tomorrow, when you go on to your ward or unit, will you worry that you don't know everything? No. So, relax; be content to learn that small part of analysis and statistics that you need to know today.

Just as with our analysis, this synthesis is something with which you can disagree. However, in order to challenge it, you must bring more evidence or demonstrate that the synthesis here has been illogically construed.

So, we analyse something by separating out its component parts in order to better understand them. We use synthesis to generate new ideas, to make new sense of the issue or phenomenon in question. This is how it is with your essays and that is exactly how it is with the analysis we see being used in research. It makes little difference whether research uses words or numbers; the data (the words or the numbers) are subject to analysis, just as the ideas in your essays are. So, you already understand analysis. When you write an essay, you question the material contained in your essay. In exactly the same way, when we collect data in research, we subject the data to questioning – that is, we analyse the data. Sometimes, research does not only tell us something we did not know before; sometimes it also helps us to build a new kind of understanding. We use this new kind of understanding to synthesise new theory. Perhaps you have already achieved this in your essays. Perhaps you have begun to add to what is already known with new ideas of your own. Such is synthesis and so it is that you may already be skilled at it.

However, just like your essays, research does not always result in a new synthesis; often we have to be content with knowing better what we already knew reasonably well before. Just like your essays really, new ideas – those that have not been thought of before – are rare and the process of producing new theory is a gradual one.

So, now you understand the fundamental and important aspects of analysis and there is just the detail to be covered, so let's do that now.

Analysing numerical data

Let's make it clear straight away that you do not need to know how to calculate a statistical analysis. In the same way, you do not need to know how a cardiac monitor produces its display or even how your MP3 player works. It works and that's all you need to know. There are people who spend their lives studying the electronics inside the MP3 player and the maths inside statistical procedures. We do not need to know why they choose to do this, but we can be pleased that we didn't make that life choice. Our happy lot is to use the tools that these people devise for us. So, you can put your paper and pencil away now. Researchers do not calculate statistical analysis with a pencil and paper; they use a computer and they use programs on the computer that have been designed to produce statistical output. These programs are like word processors for numbers.

Statistical analysis is analysis; it is used to help us clarify the nature of the data and to find things that might be hidden in the data, to find new information that is not clear without the analysis. For this to be successful, we need to know what it is that we want to find out. This is very similar to the problem-solving used in the nursing process. Before we work out what intervention is needed, we have to identify the problem. In analysis of numerical data, we need to be just as focused and just as clear about what it is we are looking for. It is not possible to run a series of randomly selected statistical analyses and then step back and see what happens.

There are two kinds of statistical procedure, descriptive and inferential. Descriptive statistics serve only to summarise data. The mean or average is a descriptive statistic, as is sum or total. In order to understand how old we are, we add up the years, so I am 52. This is my total, the sum of my years. One simple but rather large number summarises all of my numbers.

Inferential statistics are designed to determine the degree to which we can be sure about the correlation or difference between sets of data. In practice, we want to know whether any difference that exists is due simply to chance or whether it is due to the effect of the variable that we think may be causing the difference (causing the effect). This is a rather long-winded way of saying that inferential statistics are all about identifying whether an effect is significant. Let us look at significance in a little more detail because it is worth under-standing this well; after all, it is the main purpose of all inferential statistical procedures to produce the level of significance.

It may come as a surprise to you to hear that statistics never prove anything. It follows that, to a large extent, science doesn't prove anything either. This may come as a surprise because most of us have a notion of science that has to do with objectivity and facts. After all, surely science is all about the discovery of known things rather than things that are about opinion and belief. In truth, statis-tics are often at the core of what we know of as science. Science is about teasing out from everything we don't know the one or two things that we might know or that we think we know. Science recognises the world as an uncertain place but tries to tease out which bits of the world we can be more certain about. Statistics deal with this uncertainty by identifying exactly how uncertain we are.

'Probability' is a word that both science and statistical analysis use to indicate the degree to which they are sure about something. However, probability reflects the fact that we never allow ourselves to be 100% certain about anything. In fact, there are a few things that we think we are certain about; these things are called laws in science. I am as certain as I can be that if I held an apple in my hand and then dropped that apple, it would drop and not float off into the atmosphere. The behaviour of my apple is pretty predictable and is related to Newton's law of gravity. So, we do think we know some things, but there are very few such laws and very few indeed that can be said to relate to nursing.

Theories are a step or two down the knowledge ladder from laws. A theory, such as psychoanalytical or Freudian theory, is a collection of closely inter-related ideas that have some empirical referents, meaning that the theory relates in at least a few ways to what we regard as known facts. However, theory is always evolving. A theory, such as psychoanalytical theory, is in fact a law that is still growing up and still making mistakes.

So, to understand both science and statistical analysis, we must appreciate that the world is a very, very uncertain place. We do know a little about our world, but there is a great deal that we still do not understand. As we apply research to push back the barriers of knowledge, our ignorance of the world takes the form of apparently chance findings. There are things, or variables, in our world that behave unpredictably, because we don't understand them fully. There are other variables of which we are not yet even aware. These partly or completely unknown variables influence our research. It sometimes seems that as soon as we think we know about variable *a*, variable *b* comes along and proves us wrong. It may even be that we don't know what variable *b* is and that for the moment we have to refer to it as 'chance'. Chance is that part of the world that we do not understand but is still active and may impact on us and on our research.

The world of science is unpredictable and changing. Although this unpre-dictability will not change while we are still so ignorant of the world, we do have a way of measuring the impact of what we don't yet know. It is this which we call 'probability'. The purpose of almost all inferential statistical analyses is the measurement of probability – that is, the measurement of the risk that the effect we are looking at may be due solely to chance. Probability informs us of the effect that unknown variables (or chance) may be having on our work.

Let us say that we have tested a new analgesic drug against a placebo. We have tested the drug by asking participants to rate their pain after taking the drug or the placebo. We now have one set of data for the placebo and one set of data for the new drug. The two sets of data look different and we suspect that the new drug has worked better than the placebo. However, we need to make sure that our result could not have occurred by chance, so that if we ran the research again we would get a different result, perhaps one that supported the placebo. So, we have run a statistical analysis on the data because we know that this will tell us the probability of the result being due to chance.

Inferential statistical procedures (statistics) are designed to produce a value for probability, which tells us what risk there is that the result of the research was due just to chance. This value is indicated by the letter p, followed by a number. Take a look at some examples here:

$p. = 0.05$ There is a 5% risk that the result is due only to chance.

$p. < 0.001$ There is a less than 1 in 1000 risk that the result is due only to chance.

Both these results could be regarded as significant. The word 'significant' is used when we think it is safe to assume that chance did not play a part in the result of the analysis. However, it is up to us (you and me) to decide what is significant. A probability of 0.05, meaning a risk of 5% (5 in 100), is generally regarded as the minimum level for significance. However, for drug trials, we might want to be much more certain that chance has had no part to play in our research.

> ## Example from practice
>
> Imagine that you are due to drive across a bridge that spans a wide, deep river. You have been told that the bridge is safe. The designers of the bridge are sure about this and their research was significant to $p = 0.05$ (5%).
>
> Would you drive across this bridge? I think that I would want that p to be a much smaller number.

Statistical analysis is a real help in determining the risk that the result of our research is due only to chance. However, it is important that we understand that the calculation of probability, and indeed research and science in general, can never, ever prove anything. We can never, ever be that certain about any of our research. Even if we have a very small p value (as in $p. < 0.0000000000001$), there will always be a 1 at the end of the zeros. That 1 is the necessary acceptance that we can never be wholly sure. It is an acceptance that we can be wrong, that we are fallible and ignorant of many of the factors that play a part in what we are seeking to research. Perhaps this is the ultimate irony for the scientific age, for indeed we have demonstrated here that we can never be sure. In searching for truths and facts about our world, we have discovered something quite disturbing: that we can never be sure about anything. This should not worry us too much. Knowing that we are uncertain means that it is important to measure that level of uncertainty in our research – that is what probability does and it is chiefly the reason for us using statistical analysis in the first place.

When your tutor tells you that your essay needs a little more analysis, he or she is really saying that your essay needs a little more of 'you' in it, more of your own thoughts, your effort to make sense of the content that you have found in books and journals. It is just the same with research: the analysis is something that goes on inside the researcher's head. Statistical procedures cannot think; rather, they are tools to help us discern what the data contain. In essence, statistical procedures tell us whether a particular finding (a result) may have occurred by chance or whether it is likely to show a true difference or correlation between groups of data.

Let's look at our imaginary research project on patient pain. Here, we had two groups of patients; both groups had pain. We gave one group an analgesic drug and we used the other group as a control – that is, we didn't give them anything. Let's say that these are the resulting data (pain scores):

Control group	Drug group
1	1
2	2
1	2
2	1
1	2
2	1
1	2
2	1
1	2
2	1
2	2
10	7
10	7
10	7
10	7
10	7
10	7
10	7
10	7
10	7
107 sum	80 sum
5.35 mean	4.0 mean
4.33 standard deviation	2.81 standard deviation
Mann–Whitney test = 159.5 (p = 0.257)[2]	

[2] SPSS version 16.

New words

Inferential statistics Literally meaning to draw inferences from the data. Inferential statistics are used to give us a measure of significance, to tell us the likelihood that a measured difference (between two groups of data) could have occurred by chance. In contrast, descriptive statistics, such as total and mean, merely describe or summarise the data.

Each patient has scored their pain on a scale of 1–10, with 1 being little or no pain and 10 being a lot of pain. If we look at the average (mean) score for each group, we see that we have a pretty conclusive result in favour of the analgesic group. This seems to show that the patients who received the analgesia experienced less pain:

Control group average pain score = 5.35

Drug group average pain score = 4.0

So there we have it: although we need a larger sample size to be certain of this effect (the result), it looks to be quite clear that giving people analgesia will reduce their pain. However, let's just look at the other numbers to make sure. The total score (sum) seems to agree with the mean scores: the control group scored higher (had more pain) than the drug group (had less pain). Now let's look at the standard deviation. This is a measure of the dispersion around the mean. This is nothing more than a technical term for how spread out the values are. Note that the standard deviation for the control group is quite large, meaning that the data are quite spread out around the mean. Look at the data for the control group: some scores are low, while others are high. The average value is 5.35; what do you think about this?

- Do we expect the mean to reflect or summarise the data?

- In this case, does the mean accurately reflect the data?

- Did any single participant (patient) give a score on or near 5.35?

The mean should reflect the data, but here it doesn't. The mean does not reflect the data because the data vary a lot. In fact, there seem to be two groups of patients in the control group – some have a lot of pain and some don't seem to have much pain. Their pain scores vary a lot – in other words, there is a high level of dispersion around the mean and, consequently, the standard deviation (which measures the dispersion around the mean) is relatively high for the control group.

Now let's look at the result for the Mann-Whitney test. This is an inferential statistical procedure, designed to show whether the difference between two groups of data could have occurred only by chance - that is, had nothing to do with whether the patients were given analgesia or not. The result from the Mann-Whitney test is 0.257. To be considered significant (not due to chance), the result would have to be less than (<) 0.05. The number we have (0.257) is much bigger than (<) 0.05. So, there is a difference between the scores given by the two groups of patients, but that difference is not significant. In other words, we have no reason to believe that the difference as represented by the mean values was related to the use or otherwise of the analgesic drug.

The Mann-Whitney procedure does what most inferential statistical procedures do: it measures the variance *within* each group of data and then it measures the variance *between* the (two) groups of data. In general:

> If the *between-groups* variance (difference between the groups of data) is greater than the *within-groups* variance, then the result will be significant.

> If the *between-groups* variance (difference between the groups of data) is less than the *within-groups* variance, then the result will be non-significant.

So, statistical procedures tell us whether a difference that exists (between two or more groups of data) is likely to be due to a chance event or to the thing that we are trying to measure.

What statistical procedures tell us about data is actually quite limited. We need to be careful how we use and how we interpret the results of statistical procedures. All the time, we need to engage our mind when looking at data and the results of any statistical analysis. Indeed, if you look at the data in our example again, you will immediately spot the problem: It is now obvious that the variation in scores within each of the two groups is not expected and this warns us that something is wrong. You have learned a lot. Now you can look at data and provide at least an educated guess at whether the result will be significant or not. Know about statistics? You already know them so well that you can anticipate what the result will be.

Using the right statistical procedure

There are a lot of statistical procedures (you may know them as statistical tests). Some procedures are appropriate in some situations and some in other situations. So, the first thing we need to know is how to choose the most appropriate statistical procedure.

> ### New words
>
> **Correlation** The word 'correlation' is similar to 'association'. We deal in correlations when we want to know whether one set of data behaves synchronously with another. Children's weights and ages do this. There are lightweight, older children and heavyweight younger children, but on the whole, as children grow older (one set of data) their weight increases (another set of data). In determining this, we do not conclude that weight and age are the same thing; they are not the same thing but these two different things (variables) are correlated.
>
> The fact that two sets of data are correlated does not mean that one variable causes the other. Weight is associated with age but being heavy does not cause one to be old.

If you are reading a research paper, you will want to check that the statistical procedures that were used were the appropriate ones. However, there is an important caveat here. If you have selected your research paper from a good-quality journal, then the paper will have been peer-reviewed. In this way, it will have been checked by someone who does not know the author. The person who did this checking will have more knowledge of statistical analysis than you are likely to have. So, what does this mean? In practice, it means that you can be fairly sure that the proper analyses were conducted and that you only really need to document (in your essay) why it was appropriate.

So, what do you need to know? Not much really, or not now anyway. It would be useful for you to know a little about how statistical procedures are chosen, so let us look at a small range of commonly used statistical procedures.

Correlations or differences?

There are two fundamentally different questions that we can ask of data: are groups of data correlated or are they different? Remember: we have to be clear and focused about what we are looking for in the data. Sometimes we want to find out whether one group of data correlates with another group of data, and sometimes we want to find out whether one group of data is different from another group of data.

We might want to know whether children's weight is correlated with their age. Of course, children's weight *does* correlate with their age. As children grow older, their weight tends to increase. This stands to reason, doesn't it? This is an important point: whatever analysis we choose should be logically derived from what we want to find out; indeed, it should always stand to reason in this way. Would we want to know whether children's weight is different from their age? No, such a question does not make sense. The questions we ask of the data should always make sense. This is always sense that absolutely anyone can understand.

Now let us think about the other main question we can ask of data: is one group of data different from another.

Let us assume that we have a sample of patients who are all in pain. We divide this sample into two groups. We give one group an analgesic drug and the other group we give no intervention.

We then ask the whole sample to tell us how much pain they have. Do we want to find out whether the two sets of data (the pain scores) are correlated? No, of course not; we want to know whether the two sets of data are different. This is often the question asked of experiments - that is, does the experimental variable (the intervention) cause an effect on the dependent variable (the pain score)?

We need to note here that different statistical procedures are used where we look for evidence of correlations and where we look for evidence of differences. We will look at some of these procedures later in this chapter, but for now let's just note that correlations and differences relate to one of the important ways in which we look at data.

Identifying the correct statistical tool: key questions to ask

New words

Univariate One variable, for example the effect of providing analgesia on pain perception.

Multivariate More than one variable, for example the effect of providing (a) an analgesic drug and (b) psychological therapy on (a) pain, (b) anxiety and (c) contentedness with treatment.

How many groups are contained in the analysis?

It is easiest to think about data analysis as just involving two groups of data. In fact, all researchers would probably like to keep to just two groups. Unfortunately, it is sometimes necessary to analyse data from more than two groups at the same time. For example, we might need to compare the effect of two analgesic drugs against a control; this would give us three groups of data. Sometimes, we know that there are lots of variables that might be causing an effect and so we need to include them all in the analysis.

There are two important considerations here. The first is that the number of groups of data will help to determine which statistical procedure we use. The second is that statistical analyses become more complex as the number of groups of data increases. No one wants this to happen; it is seriously undesirable. An analysis should always teach us something new about the data; it should never confuse us. Laboratory researchers will go to great lengths to reduce the number of variables with which they have to deal at any one time. They will ensure that they have only one chemical in their test tube and not a mix of chemicals. Unfortunately, those of us who wish to research human beings often find that we can't squash them into test tubes: they usually won't fit and they are rarely willing to be put in one anyway. All too often, we are interested in the complex mix of variables that is human life, and so our analyses tend to be multivariate, composed of several or even many variables.

What is the level of measurement?

This is easy: we have already worked it out. We have noted that numerical data exist within one of three levels of measurement. We noted that each of these levels of measurement has a separate collection of statistical procedures associated with them. These are:

- nominal (categories);

- ordinal (items placed in order or any short scale);

- interval or ratio[3] (a long scale).

Is the design related or unrelated?

This is the last question we need to ask, at least for the range of statistical procedures that we will be looking at here. A related design is one where the data are collected from the same sample of people (here, we are usually dealing with people) on more than one occasion. So, it will be clear now that an unrelated design is where the researcher collects data from two or more different groups of people. We do not need to ask this question when correlations are being looked for because correlational designs are always related and, in any case, they have their own range of statistical procedures.

---

[3] When it comes to numerical analysis, interval and ratio data are treated similarly.

It is probably the case that more research designs in nursing are of the unrelated kind. When we determined the effect of providing an analgesic to patients in pain, we had two groups; one group was given an analgesic drug and the other was not provided with any intervention. Those two groups of people were different people; they didn't even know each other. If we had used a before-after design, we might have put both groups of people together and then measured their pain before and after giving them (all) the analgesic drug. In this last situation, we would have a related design.

Related designs tend to be longitudinal in quality, with data being collected from the same people on more than one occasion. With unrelated designs, data are collected from two or more different groups of people at more or less the same time.

How many groups or conditions are there?

In Chapter 3, we saw that different research designs produce a different number of groups of data. A survey, for example, often contains just one group of data. We might stop people in the street and ask them what they think of the NHS. We might want to sample older people in this particular study. So, we would have one big group of older people in a study. We might not want to compare them with any other group of people; we might only be interested in the views of older people. In this example, we have just one group.

Often, we want to compare one condition with another. Perhaps we want to compare the effects of two drugs. In this case, we will have at least two conditions, represented by the data that we receive from patients who were given drug *a* and drug *b*.

The number of conditions contained within a research design is one factor that we need to take into account when choosing the most appropriate statistical procedure. For example, a t test can be used to compare two groups (conditions), but for more than two groups we will need to use a form of analysis of variance (ANOVA). Don't worry about these statistical procedures just now.

You can now select the appropriate statistical procedure

It will have occurred to you by now that we have been looking at statistics without actually mentioning many of them by name. This is because statistical procedures all do pretty much the same job, but there are different procedures (different statistics) for different kinds of data and where we want to ask differ-ent questions about the data, for example whether the data contain correlations or differences.

With the help of Figure 6.1, you are now able to select the appropriate statisti-cal procedure for a range of commonly used research designs. Even if some of this chapter has been a little difficult to grasp, you do now have the skills to select the right statistical procedure from quite a range of statistics that will fill a whole page. Take a quick look at Figure 6.1, be suitably awestruck and then read on to discover that you already do understand how to select the right statistical procedure for a variety of research designs.

In 1 minute you will have:

- been horrified by the number of statistical procedures available;
- decided that it is too complex for anyone to understand.

In 2 more minutes you will have:

- demonstrated to yourself that you do understand it and that you can select appropriate statistical procedures for a variety of research designs.

Now look at Figure 6.1 and select the most appropriate statistical procedure for the following research designs:

Design 1

This study looks at the difference in regard for the NHS between a sample of people aged 20-30 years and a sample of people aged 65-85 years. The par-ticipants are asked 'Do you trust the NHS to care for you when you are ill?' The participants are asked to answer simply 'yes', 'no' or 'not sure'.

The data produced by this study are *nominal* (the categories are 'yes', 'no' and 'not sure').

It is hypothesised that there will be *differences* between the responses from the younger and the older group of participants.

The design is *unrelated* because the two groups of participants have nothing to do with each other (the design would be related if the study asked younger people about the NHS and then waited until years later, when they had aged and become older people, before asking them the same question again).

Common statistical procedure

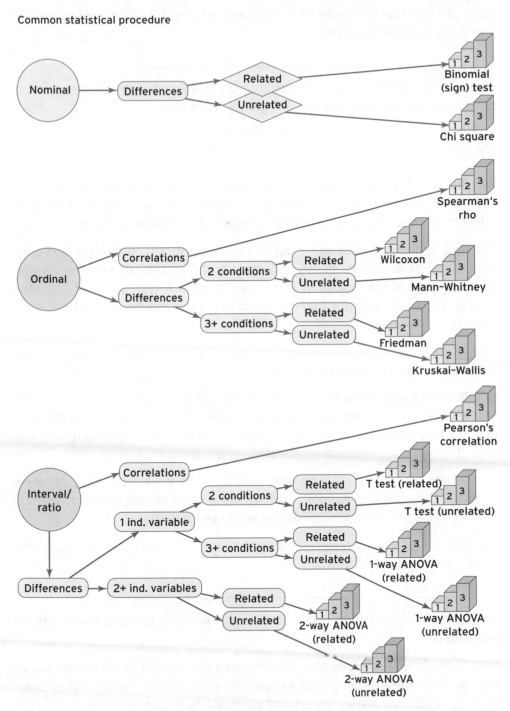

Figure 6.1 Selecting the appropriate statistical procedure

Look at Figure 6.1 and write here the name of the statistical procedure that should be used for this study:

_____

Correct! You did it: it is chi square. Let's do that again with something much more complicated (I am sure you will get this right too).

Design 2

We want to run an experiment to see whether anti-hypertensive drugs, increased exercise or both anti-hypertensive drugs and increased exercise have the best effect on the blood pressure of people being treated for hypertension.

The data collected by the study will be blood-pressure recordings. Blood pressure will be measured in mmHg on a scale that (theoretically) can be zero (or less) and that is continuous (it is possible to have a systolic BP of 120.3456 mmHg, should we wish for that degree of accuracy). So the level of measurement is *interval/ratio*.

The study hypothesises that there will be *differences* between the data collected from the three groups of patients.

In this experiment, there is *one independent variable* – the type of treatment. This independent variable has *three conditions* – the three groups of patients, i.e. anti-hypertensive drugs, increased exercise and increased exercise together with anti-hypertensive drugs.

The design of the study will be *unrelated* because we will be using different people for the three conditions (if we used the same people, exposing them to each condition in turn, then the design would be related).

So, look at Figure 6.1 and write here the name of the statistical procedure that should be used for this study:

_____

Awesome! The most appropriate statistical procedure is the one-way ANOVA (unrelated).

Well done! So statistics are easy. The research design tells us which one to use. We run that one-way analysis of variance (unrelated) in a statistics application such as SPSS® just like we use a word processor to process words.

In 1 minute you have:

- been horrified by the number of statistical procedures available; ✓
- decided that it is too complex for anyone to understand. ✓

In 2 more minutes you have:

- proved to yourself that you do understand it and that you can select appropriate statistical procedures for a variety of research designs. ✓

What does a one-way analysis of variance do? It does what all inferential statistical procedures do: it looks at whether the within-group variance is greater or less than the between-group variance (whether the difference in BP scores *between* the three groups of hypertensive patients is greater or less than the degree to which the scores *within* each group vary). In doing this, it will tell us to what degree we can be sure that any difference between the groups is due to the effect of the independent variable or whether we should deduce that any such difference is due merely to chance. The one-way analysis of variance will give us a probability value (p), which will tell us what risk there is that any differences between the groups is due just to chance. If you understand the meaning of the p value in a one-way analysis of variance, you understand its meaning in all inferential statistical procedures.

Qualitative analysis

Qualitative data usually exist in the form of words, but they can take the form of images, video or historical data. Recordings of the spoken word are usually transcribed before they are made subject to analysis. While quantitative analysis usually seeks to count the data, qualitative analysis seeks to find meaning in the data. In this way, a qualitative analysis seeks to find the same meaning or interpretation of the data that other people would find if they undertook the analysis. In this way, the analysis of qualitative data achieves a level of objectivity. In practice, qualitative analysis is both objective and systematic. However, qualitative analysis can seem relatively easy to understand; it can seem 'soft' and 'friendly'. This is largely because the data (usually in the form of words) are reported using normal language, making the data much more readily understandable than statistics in quantitative studies.

Here is an excerpt from the qualitative analysis of data from Fernandez and Wilson's (2008) study on Maori mothers' smoking habits. The researchers identified themes that were common to the interview data. Here, we offer an example of the theme 'being a mother'. In this way, being a mother is suggested as one factor that influenced the Maori women to stop smoking.

> Motherhood had special significance for participants. Being a mother was particularly significant during their experiences of pregnancy, and in response to positive feelings about their children. Their babies' health was consequently identified as being important. Therefore, quitting or not smoking during pregnancy was perceived as maternal acts of protecting and nurturing their unborn babies. Some participants acknowledged their gratitude to their babies for 'making' them quit:
>
> *'I always give up when I'm pregnant' (Participant A).*
>
> *'I thank my baby; she made me give up smoking' (Participant B).*
>
> Participants also agreed that apart from their own health, their children were the most important reason for them to stay smoke-free:
>
> *'Health has kept me motivated [to stay smoke-free] and my kids' (Participant E).*
>
> *Fernandez and Wilson (2008, p. 32)*

You can see that the results of qualitative analyses such as this are immediately understandable. This is because the analysis is expressed in the same language as the data. Indeed, it is important to the qualitative researchers that the participants themselves would at least understand and agree with the themes drawn from their own transcript.

The apparent simplicity of qualitative results often serves to endear this form of research to people who don't have a background in statistics (most of us). However, not understanding statistics is not a good reason to use qualitative research. Qualitative research has a particular function in exploring meaning in the human world. However, qualitative research cannot be used in every aspect of research. Furthermore, qualitative analysis can take much longer than a typical quantitative analysis. Imagine undertaking 12 interviews, each lasting just one hour. It could easily take a day to transcribe every one of those 12 interviews. At this point, the data still need coding, something that will take at least two people perhaps many hours. Themes such as the one illustrated above will then need to be identified, and all of this will need verifying with another person and perhaps with the participants. The extraction of codes and themes from textual data is a task that often takes a great deal of time.

Notwithstanding the above, qualitative research as it is published in the professional journals can indeed be easy to understand. There are no numbers and the results are expressed in the language we use every day. This can be a positive advantage if you are having to write an essay on research or evidence-based practice, when qualitative research can indeed make the task a more pleasant one.

New words

Raw data Data as they have been collected and before they have been analysed.

Bear in mind that just as with a statistical analysis of quantitative data, the analysis must be rigorous, systematic and objective. Qualitative research is real research in every way that is important. Perhaps the only difference is that qualitative research is research on the participants who took part in the study. It is not usually possible to make inferences about the larger population in the way that quantitative research often claims to be able to do. In this way, Fernandez and Wilson's (2008) study on Maori women's smoking behaviour should be considered to be about only those women in the study. The relationship between what we know of these women and what we may think we know of Maori women in general is much less clear than it might be in a quantitative study. Qualitative researchers often seek to make no claim on how their data might be reflective of a wider population. This in no way limits the worth of qualitative research, not least because in its favour qualitative research can elicit and expose material of much greater depth than is usually possible in quantitative research. Qualitative research offers the opportunity to really explore people's attitudes, feelings and experiences in a way and to a depth that is hardly possible in quantitative research.

Let's look at how a typical qualitative researcher might go about analysing their data. The raw data will usually be in the form of interviews recorded on tape or disk.

Transcription of the data

The first step is to transcribe the data so that they exist in an electronic format, as words in a word-processor file.

Coding of the data

This is a process where similar text is given the same code (the code can be any-thing, such as a, b, c ... or more meaningful labels can be used). What exactly is coded will depend on what is being looked for. Sometimes the researcher will have a predetermined (sometimes called 'a priori') set of ideas and will know what he or she is looking for even before reading the transcripts. More usually, what is found and coded in the transcript will develop from what is found there and the researcher will try to have no predetermined view on what should be found in the transcripts (these codes are said to be grounded in the data). In this case, especially, coding can be a lengthy process. The codes are continually refined, because they are being built up in real time. In this way, whenever a code is assigned to a piece of text, all the other pieces of text already assigned that code will be reviewed in order to make sure that the code in use continues to reflect the same meaning in the text. It may become apparent that two mean-ings are present and that a single code has to be re-fashioned into two codes in order to properly reflect the meaning in the transcript.

Developing themes

The increasing collection of codes is then sorted into meaningful categories or themes. Such themes might be 'pain', 'fear', 'family', 'recovery', etc. In this way, each theme will exist as a kind of overarching collection of codes. Usually, these themes are built up and developed as the transcripts are read and coded. The process is dynamic; that is, the process of developing the codes and themes is one that involves a continuous interaction with the data. As one transcript is being read, the researcher is continuously referring back to tran-scripts that have already been read. This process continues until all the transcripts have been read and the researcher is happy that both the codes and the themes fully reflect the meaning that exists in all of the transcripts. This may sound like a very time-consuming process. It is.

New words

Validity Validity means 'truth'. In research, it is the degree to which the data has been interpreted as they were understood by the participant who provided the data.

Reliability The degree to which a second analysis of the data would agree with the first analysis.

Validity and reliability

The process so far may sound like little more than the expression of the researcher's opinion on what is contained in the transcripts. Indeed, it is the case that the researcher does interact with the data and, in a way, the researcher and his or her ideas and values do become part of the analysis. There are three main ways in which qualitative analysis deals with this issue:

- It is simply accepted that the researcher is part of the analysis. In this way, the researcher becomes embedded in the research. This can be done, for example, when researchers live and work with the participants, as in social anthropological studies.

- The coding is also conducted by at least one other individual. It is then possible to demonstrate the inter-coder reliability, or the degree to which the two (or more) coders have agreed.

- The coding of the transcripts and the themes that have been drawn from the transcripts can be taken back to the participants. In this way, the participants are asked whether the themes appropriately reflect what they said or meant to say.

In addition, it is common to find that researchers include quotations in their research reports that are meant to give credence to the themes generated from the data. We have already seen this in Fernandez and Wilson's (2008) study. Such quotations also make the research report somewhat easier to understand.

Validity and reliability are terms that can be a little difficult to relate to qualitative research. Nevertheless, qualitative research should make clear the methods that were used to enable the analysis to be convincing. In practice, there is an almost unending and constantly evolving number of such mechanisms, which makes qualitative research rather less cut and dried than quantitative research. This should not matter; what does matter is that each study should include a justification of the form of analysis used. It is then, rightfully, for the reader to be convinced or otherwise. Qualitative research is not for those who like to be constrained by rules and regulations. This freedom from set methods and a willingness instead to be embedded in the data is surely one of the strengths of qualitative research.

Concluding remarks

Data analysis of any kind exists to serve two purposes. The first purpose of analysis is to discover things (effects) within the data, effects that might not be at all obvious from looking at the raw data (sometimes called 'eyeballing the data'). This is exactly the same mechanism that you employ when you apply analysis to the discussion in your essay. The second purpose is to summarise the data in order to make them more understandable and to make it possible to communicate the data in a way that will be both succinct and meaningful. However, even the most complex statistical analysis is only a tool. Analysis does not remove from the researcher the responsibility to consider the data carefully and to critically evaluate what the analysis has shown, together with any weaknesses inherent in that analysis. As professionals who may be asked to integrate research findings into practice, nurses are free to criticise an analysis and to suggest alternative interpretations of the data.

Data analysis, especially when it is quantitative and statistical, probably does scare many people away from research. However, we have seen here that data analysis really can be easy to understand. We should bear in mind that no one knows everything about data analysis and that even the most accomplished researchers tend to be familiar only with the kinds of analysis used in their own field of work. Of course, there are many forms of data analysis that have not been covered in this chapter, but the principles of data analysis, as those principles affect almost any kind of data, have indeed been covered here. That's a great start and one that will allow you to develop your understanding further.

Summary

- A knowledge of mathematics is not needed. Researchers use computer applications, not a pencil and paper.

- Inferential statistical procedures (tests) do not prove anything; rather, they demonstrate the degree to which chance may have had an effect on the research.

- It is up to you and me to decide whether the level of probability (as in $p = 0.05$) is acceptable. We are free to suggest that a higher level of significance would be desirable.

- Selecting the correct statistical procedure is not usually difficult, even though there are many statistical procedures available.

- Qualitative analysis is a resource-heavy and often time-consuming process, but it produces an analysis that is both thorough and relatively easy to understand.

- In general, the purpose of any analysis is to summarise the data and to extract from the data information that is often not otherwise readily apparent.

Further reading

A great way to learn more about statistical analysis is to explore the computer application known as SPSS. This is an expensive product but most universities make it available to students. SPSS originally stood for Statistical Package for the Social Sciences. More information on the SPSS suite of applications can be found at **www.spss.com**.

SPSS is shipped with some example data files; your university computer centre will show you where to find these. Try loading in some data and simply play with the application.

There are several good books that can help you get to grips with SPSS and with quantitative data analysis, including these:

Pallant, J. (2007). *SPSS Survival Manual: A Step by Step Guide to Data Analysis Using SPSS for Windows*. Milton Keynes: Open University Press.

Field, A. (2005). *Discovering Statistics Using SPSS*. London: Sage Publications Limited.

The following is a guide to actually undertaking qualitative research. The text, though, is unusual in offering a relatively straightforward and practical account of qualitative research:

Silverman, D. (2004). *Doing Qualitative Research: A Practical Handbook*. London: Sage Publications Limited.

References

Fernandez, C. and D. Wilson (2008) 'Maori women's views on smoking cessation initiatives'. *Nursing Praxis in New Zealand* **24**(2): 27-40.

Chapter 7
How to succeed with your essay on research and evidence-based practice

Most nursing programmes contain a module on evidence-based practice or research. This book was written because many students find research to be difficult to understand. The real test of that understanding is the essay that many students have to write on the subject. Of course, such modules and courses vary in what they demand of students. However, many students find themselves having to review one or more research papers or to examine the evidence that supports an aspect of practice. Students should always get advice first of all from their own module tutors. However, this chapter contains some general advice on how to write a capable essay.

The assessment is set because your faculty recognises the importance of research in nursing and wants you to be able to understand research and to be able to use it in your practice. However, there are one or two difficulties that are inherent in an assessment of this kind. First, your faculty staff would probably prefer you to get some experience in real-life research. This is not usually possible because it would take too long, there isn't enough research going on to provide the experience and nursing cohorts are simply too large. It is because of this that your faculty may decide to ask you to review a piece of research or to look at the degree to which an aspect of practice is supported by evidence. This seems reasonable enough, until one realises that students are being asked to critique or evaluate something of which they have no experience. In this respect, it is like being asked to tell someone how to drive a car when you have never sat in one yourself.

So, it is not that research is complex or difficult to understand. It is not complex and it is not difficult to understand. The issue here is that you have probably never been involved in any research. However, nursing is developing and it is not yet perfect; while it is still imperfect, there will be challenges to face.

Unfortunately, what we have discussed so far is not the only issue. These assessments are not only difficult to write; they are also difficult to mark. There are two broad ways in which an examiner can regard your essay:

- How well your essay works as an essay.

- How well you have understood the research.

In the second of the two categories, there may be an expectation that emphasises the research design and methodology or one that emphasises the analysis. In any case, what is expected of you should be identified very clearly in your module or course handbook. If you are still unclear about what is expected of you, ask someone. It can also be useful to get together with other students who are keen to do well with this assessment, meet several times and work things out together. If you are all still unclear about what is being required of you, go and see the module leader and don't leave his or her office until you have a clear explanation of what is required (you may need to take sandwiches).

Tips on writing a good essay on research and evidence-based practice

Some students enjoy studying and others prefer to pick up their knowledge as they go along. Student nurses on placement, however, are rather unlikely to become involved in research and so research is something that benefits from a reasonable amount of reading. The more you read about research, the more you will become familiar with the language of research. You will then be able to use this language in your essay and it will be clear to the examiner that you are familiar with and comfortable with the language of research. This is time-consuming and needs to be built into your busy schedule. This is one essay that should not be left to the last moment.

> Read about research. This is time-consuming and needs to be built into your busy schedule. This is one essay that should not be left to the last moment.

Just as you should try to become familiar with the language of research, it helps a lot if you can become familiar with the clinical issue that you will discuss. So, for example, you may want to write your essay about the research on postoperative pain. In this case, make sure you know about postoperative pain. After all, you will want to introduce the subject of postoperative pain in your essay and your conclusion will be about postoperative pain. A lot of your essay will actually be about postoperative pain, so become familiar with it as a subject. This will also help you to understand the research. If you are able to, you can save yourself a lot of time by choosing to look at the research available on an aspect of practice with which you are already familiar.

> Become familiar with the clinical issue that you will discuss.

Try to be up to date with your general essay-writing skills. This is no time to have to struggle with that as well. If this isn't possible, make sure that at least you reference properly. Get a copy of your faculty's referencing guidelines, read those guidelines and stick to them. Good referencing is often considered to be more important in the field of research, and the examiner may expect that that is reflected in your essay.

> Make sure that you reference properly.

It may be that you have written all of your previous essays without obtaining any tutorial help. You may be nervous about asking a tutor to critique your work. However, this is one essay on which help is decidedly useful. Go and see your tutor as soon as possible, at the beginning of the module, find out what help he or she is able to offer and then use that help. Your tutor will guide you about what you need to include in your essay and will help to explain some of those research terms. Be brave: see your tutor and ask for feedback on your essay. Use whatever resources your faculty makes available to you.

> Go and see your tutor as soon as possible, find out what help he or she is able to offer and then use that help.

Understand that your research critique is an exercise in communication, just like every other essay you have written. Your essay should tell a story and have a beginning, a middle and an end. Your essay should be about something and have a clearly transparent purpose. It can be useful to ask yourself what you are trying to communicate and why.

> Your essay should be about something and have a clearly transparent purpose.

Your essay should be in three parts:

1. An introduction (discussion)

2. A review of the research (description)

3. A discussion of the implications of the research (analysis).

> Your essay should be in three parts: An introduction, a review, a discussion.

In the introduction, consider including two pieces of discussion. The first should be about the need and purpose of research in nursing and health care. The second should introduce the clinical problem (the focus of the research, such as postoperative pain).

If you are reviewing research, make sure that you include some discussion on:

- the need for the research and the background to it;

- the design and methodology of the research – that is, how it was done;

- what the research found: don't shy away from the statistical analysis – it is important that you are able to say what the research actually found.

> Make sure that you include some discussion on the need for the research, the design and methodology, what the research found.

You may have been asked to select a piece of research on which to base your essay. You may think it best to go to a relatively easy-to-understand journal, but this may not be such a good idea. You may not be confident in differentiating a good study from a poor one. Instead, get your study from an academic journal; at least then you can be reasonably sure that the research will be of good quality. Knowing that a study is likely to be of good quality will help enormously when it comes to critiquing it. Should your chosen study have used regression analysis? If your chosen study came from a reputable academic journal, then it is very unlikely that the researchers will have chosen an inappropriate analysis. You can be reasonably sure that the regression analysis was the right thing to do. Now all you need to do is to look up regression analysis to get a definition of it that you can understand.

> Get your study from an academic journal.

By now, you will be used to critiquing things. Your faculty staff have encouraged you to question everything and to avoid being descriptive. However, you should question and critique only material that you understand. Imagine someone took you into theatre and you were able to watch a world-renowned neurosurgeon operate on someone's brain. After the operation was over, they took you to one side and said, 'Now, how well do you think they did that operation and what could they have done better?' Doubtless you would think that an odd question. So it is with research, except that your assignment may actually ask you to evaluate a piece of research. This is one occasion when it may be safer to stick to description. There is a danger that in critiquing the research, you may simply succeed in exposing your own

> Question and critique only material that you understand.

lack of knowledge. It is probably the case that the research has been carried out appropriately and that the researchers themselves have identified what weaknesses and limitations there may be in the research. Remember that in any good journal, the research paper will have been peer-reviewed by at least one person and probably two people with research and academic experience. So, be careful about critiquing the study and be prepared to be a little more descriptive than you are with your other essays. You can balance this descriptiveness by putting argument and analysis into the discussion section of your essay. The discussion section will be where you look at the implications of the research for nursing and health care, for patients and for future research. Here you can relate the research and its findings to practice and question and critique as much as you wish.

It may be that you find a research study that seems not to be perfect and you are confident that you understand it well enough to provide a critique. Even here, you should pause and consider whether the problems with the research were due to the researchers' error. It is often the case that a more perfect or more robust design and method would be fine in theory but impossible to conduct in practice. Nursing research often deals with human participants who will not readily fit in to the best research methodologies. Ethical issues, such as the need to obtain informed consent and to ensure that participants are not harmed by the research, do often limit what can be done. It is the case, for example, that very little clinical research is undertaken on the use of drugs in babies and children. This is because it is often impossible to obtain their informed consent. In the same way, research that does take place in nursing is often subject to design limitations. If you can show your understanding of these issues, rather than simply criticising the study for not being perfect, then you will have shown that you have a broad understanding of research issues.

> Consider whether the problems with the research were due to the researchers' error. It is often the case that a more perfect or more robust design and method would be fine in theory but impossible to conduct in practice.

Keep your essay simple. Research terminology is difficult enough to get to grips with, and the whole subject may be new to you. Keep it simple: do not be afraid to use language with which you are familiar rather than research language that you may not fully understand. If you make the mistake of using terminology with which you lack confidence, your lack of confidence will come across very clearly in your essay. Be content to use plain English and allow yourself to acclimatise to research terminology at your own pace.

> Keep it simple: do not be afraid to use language with which you are familiar rather than research language.

Research ethics is an important subject. It may be that you have been asked specifically to write about ethics. However, unless you have been asked specifically to write about ethics, consider not allocating too much space to a critique of the ethics.

> Unless you have been asked specifically to write about ethics, consider not allocating too much space to a critique of the ethics.

The reason for this is that authors often don't have much space to discuss ethics within the limited word count that most journals specify. In practice, it is safe to assume that their research will have been processed by a properly appointed ethics committee. It is good to mention research ethics in your essay, but do not expect there to be a full account of the ethical issues in the research paper that you are critiquing.

Lastly but importantly, be positive: show your enthusiasm for nursing and for nursing research. Nursing research and evidence-based practice are not yet perfect, but it is important to be able to deal with the diffi-

> Be positive: show your enthusiasm for nursing and for nursing research.

culties and have the enthusiasm and commitment to see how it can be improved. Remember: you are the future of nursing and the examiner will want to see that you are enthusiastic about your profession.

You will meet nurses whose only concerns are the here and nows of their present shift, their ward or area. There will probably be times when the here and now of busy practice will be your chief concern too. However, the professional nurse also possesses a responsibility to the whole profession and to the care of patients in the future. Research is not without its difficulties, but it is a necessary endeavour for nursing to progress and to improve. This book has been written to help students get both their feet firmly on the first two to three rungs of the ladder that is research in nursing. However, it isn't enough to understand research. At some point in your career you should become actively involved in research, so that you can play your part in the progress that nursing must make in order to continue to provide patients with the care they need. You *are* amazing. Enjoy the challenge!

Index